Introduction to Drug Metabolism

THIRD EDITION

G. Gordon Gibson PhD
Professor of Molecular Toxicology
School of Biomedical and Life Sciences
University of Surrey, England

Paul Skett Fil. Dr.
Senior Lecturer in Pharmacology
University of Glasgow, Scotland

First edition published in 1986 by:
Chapman & Hall
Second edition published in 1994

Third edition published in 2001 by:
Nelson Thornes Publishers
Delta Place
27 Bath Road
Cheltenham
GL53 7TH
United Kingdom

02 03 04 05 / 10 9 8 7 6 5 4 3

A catalogue record for this book is available from the British Library

ISBN 0 7487 6011 3

The cover shows a partial view of the docking of carbamazepine with the active site
of CYP3A4. Courtesy of Dr Dave Lewis, School of Biomedical and Life Sciences,
University of Surrey, England.

Every effort has been made to contact copyright holders of any material
reproduced within the text and the authors and publishers apologise if any have
been overlooked

Typeset by Aarontype Limited, Easton, Bristol
Printed and bound in Spain by GraphyCems

CONTENTS

INTRODUCTION

It is now seven years since the Second Edition of *Introduction to Drug Metabolism* was published and such has been the rapid increase in our knowledge in this area that the current Third Edition is now warranted.

The text still retains its original aim of being a primer in drug metabolism for advanced undergraduate classes in science, medicine, dentistry and pharmacy, and additionally for postgraduate students new to the area of drug metabolism and scientists in the pharmaceutical and chemical industries. The original impetus for writing this text is still of relevance today in the Third Edition, in that there is no comparative text of which we are aware that fulfils the need for an all-encompassing primer to drug metabolism, without recourse to advanced and specialised monographs and reviews. However, where relevant, we have included specific reference to these in the updated reading lists that follow each chapter, in addition to relevant web sites.

The general layout and format is essentially unchanged from the Second Edition as this was well received and we do not believe in tampering with something that is apparently working well. However, the content has been substantially changed and updated in detail to reflect the large strides made in our understanding of the subject in recent years, particularly in the areas of:

- enzymology and molecular genetics of the drug metabolising enzymes
- substantial focus on human enzymes throughout the text
- drug- and chemical-dependent regulation of the drug metabolising enzymes
- genetic polymorphisms and drug responses in the human population
- clinical relevance of the subject
- toxicological implications of drug biotransformation reactions
- substantially updated further reading lists
- addition of informative web sites on the subject.

The expertise of the two authors is complementary, with one based on biochemistry, molecular biology and toxicology (G.G.G.) and the other on pharmacology, physiology and medicine (P.S.), as is reflected in the current balanced approach to the subject.

We are indebted to our many colleagues in academia and the pharmaceutical industry and former students for comments on the Second Edition and for suggestions for its improvement, which we believe has substantially improved the Third Edition. In particular, we extend a special 'thank you' to Professors Brian Burchell and John Hayes and Dr Mike Coughtrie (all from the University of Dundee at Ninewells Hospital in Scotland) for their valuable comments and suggestions for some sections on enzymology and to Catherine Shaw and her colleagues at Nelson Thornes for their support and faith in the project. It is up to you, the reader, to determine how successful our collective efforts have been.

1 PATHWAYS OF DRUG METABOLISM

LEARNING OBJECTIVES

At the end of this chapter, you should be able to:
- List the chemical reactions involved in drug metabolism/biotransformation
- Define phase 1 and phase 2 reactions and the respective roles of the two phases of metabolism
- Characterise each reaction as a phase 1 or phase 2 reaction
- Describe each chemical reaction in terms of a full chemical equation including any co-factors involved
- Describe the synthesis of any required co-factors for the reactions
- Assess how any chemical *may* be metabolised using knowledge of the reactions above
- Discuss the relationship between endogenous metabolism and drug metabolism

1.1 INTRODUCTION

The routes by which drugs may be metabolised or biotransformed are many and varied and include oxidation, reduction, hydrolysis, hydration, conjugation and condensation reactions. It is important that these pathways are understood, as the route of metabolism of a drug can determine its ultimate pharmacological or toxicological activity. Drug metabolism is normally divided into two phases: phase 1 (or functionalisation reactions) and phase 2 (or conjugative reactions). The chemical reactions normally associated with phase 1 and phase 2 drug metabolism are given in Table 1.1.

The reactions of phase 1 are thought to act as a preparation of the drug for the phase 2 reactions, i.e. phase 1 'functionalises' the drug by producing or uncovering

Table 1.1 Reactions classed as phase 1 or phase 2 metabolism

Phase 1	Phase 2
Oxidation	Glucuronidation/glucosidation
Reduction	Sulfation
Hydrolysis	Methylation
Hydration	Acetylation
Dethioacetylation	Amino acid conjugation
Isomerisation	Glutathione conjugation Fatty acid conjugation Condensation

a chemically reactive functional group on which the phase 2 reactions can occur. Thus, the phase 2 reactions are the true 'detoxification' pathways and give products that account for the bulk of the inactive, excreted products of a drug. Many of the reactions of both phase 1 and phase 2 are capable of being performed on the same compound and, thus, there is a possibility of interaction of the various metabolic routes in terms of competing reactions for the same substrate.

This chapter will examine the different types of reactions involved in drug metabolism using the phase 1 and 2 classification as a basis. Examples of each type of reaction will be given and, where possible, these will be actual reactions of clinically relevant drug substrates rather than model substrates. This will show the pharmacological, toxicological and clinical relevance of the reactions. Attention will be drawn to competing reactions for the same substrate, where appropriate.

There is a close relationship between the biotransformation of drugs and the normal biochemical processes occurring in the body and many of the enzymes involved in drug metabolism are, in fact, principally involved in the metabolism of endogenous compounds and only metabolise drugs because the drugs closely resemble the natural compound. A separate section of this chapter will be devoted to the metabolism of endogenous compounds by 'drug metabolising' enzymes to illustrate this overlap.

In the limited space available, it is only possible to give a flavour of the range of reactions involved in drug biotransformation. It would be impossible to list every reaction undergone by every drug and inevitably there will be omissions. It is not the intention to show how every drug is metabolised but how, based on the structure of the drug, the possible metabolic routes can be discerned. Information regarding specific drugs should be sought in specialist publications. A list of further reading material will be found at the end of each chapter from which further information on specific pathways can be obtained.

1.2 PHASE 1 METABOLISM

Phase 1 metabolism includes oxidation, reduction, hydrolysis and hydration reactions, as well as other rarer miscellaneous reactions. The classification of phase 1 reactions can be found in Table 1.2. Oxidations performed by the microsomal mixed-function oxidase system (cytochrome P450-dependent) is considered separately because of its importance and the diversity of reactions performed by this enzyme system.

Table 1.2 Sub-classification of phase 1 reactions

Oxidation involving cytochrome P450
Oxidation – others
Reduction
Hydrolysis
Hydration
Isomerisation
Miscellaneous

1.2.1 Oxidations involving cytochrome P450 (the microsomal mixed-function oxidase)

The mixed-function oxidase system found in microsomes (endoplasmic reticulum) of many cells (notably those of liver, kidney, lung and intestine) performs many different functionalisation reactions (summarised in Table 1.3). All of these

Table 1.3 Reactions performed by the microsomal mixed-function oxidase system

Reaction	Substrate
Aromatic hydroxylation	Lignocaine
Aliphatic hydroxylation	Pentobarbitone
Epoxidation	Benzo[a]pyrene
N-Dealkylation	Diazepam
O-Dealkylation	Codeine
S-Dealkylation	6-Methylthiopurine
Oxidative deamination	Amphetamine
N-Oxidation	3-Methylpyridine 2-Acetylaminofluorene
S-Oxidation	Chlorpromazine
Phosphothionate oxidation	Parathion
Dehalogenation	Halothane
Alcohol oxidation	Ethanol

reactions require the presence of molecular oxygen and NADPH as well as the complete mixed-function oxidase system (cytochrome P450, NADPH-cytochrome P450 reductase and lipid). All reactions involve the initial insertion of a single oxygen atom into the drug molecule. A subsequent rearrangement and/or decomposition of this product may occur, leading to the final products seen. The mechanism of insertion of this single oxygen atom is discussed at length in Chapter 2. An example of each reaction is given below.

(i)   *Aromatic hydroxylation.* This is a very common reaction for drugs and xenobiotics containing an aromatic ring. In this example (Figure 1.1) the local anaesthetic and antidysrhythmic drug, lignocaine, is converted to its 3-hydroxy derivative.

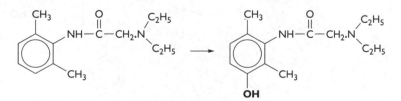

Figure 1.1 The 3-hydroxylation of lignocaine.

(ii) *Aliphatic hydroxylation.* Another very common reaction, e.g. pentobarbitone hydroxylated in the pentyl side chain (Figure 1.2).

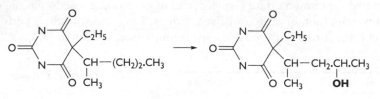

Figure 1.2 The side-chain hydroxylation of pentobarbitone.

(iii) *Epoxidation.* Epoxides are normally unstable intermediates but may be stable enough to be isolated from polycyclic compounds (e.g. the precarcinogenic polycyclic hydrocarbons). Epoxides are substrates of epoxide hydrolase (discussed later), forming dihydrodiols, but they may also spontaneously decompose to form hydroxylated products or quinones. It has been suggested that epoxide formation is the first step in aromatic hydroxylation. Figure 1.3 shows the epoxidation of benzo(a)pyrene to its 4,5-epoxide.

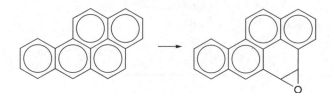

Figure 1.3 The formation of benzo[a]pyrene-4,5-epoxide.

(iv) *Dealkylation.* This reaction occurs very readily with drugs containing a secondary or tertiary amine, an alkoxy group or an alkyl substituted thiol. The alkyl group is lost as the corresponding aldehyde. The reactions are often referred to as *N*-, *O*- or *S*-dealkylations, depending on the type of atom the alkyl group is attached to. In the example of *N*-demethylation in Figure 1.4, diazepam is converted to *N*-desmethyldiazepam with the loss of methanal (formaldehyde).

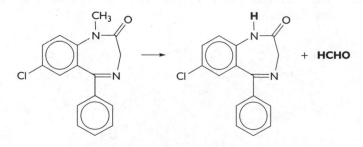

Figure 1.4 The *N*-demethylation of diazepam.

The reaction is considered to occur in two steps, the first being hydroxylation of the methyl group on the nitrogen, and the second a decomposition of this intermediate (see Figure 1.5).

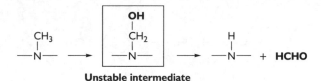

Unstable intermediate

Figure 1.5 The mechanism of N-demethylation of diazepam.

Figure 1.6 shows the O-demethylation of codeine to yield morphine. The reaction proceeds via a hydroxy intermediate as N-dealkylation.

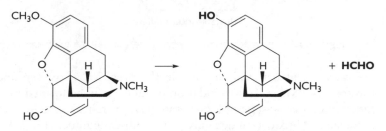

Figure 1.6 The O-demethylation of codeine.

Various S-methyl compounds can be S-demethylated. The S-demethylation of S-methylthiopurine is illustrated in Figure 1.7. The S-demethylation of 2-methylthiobenzothiazole has been reported, however, to require glutathione and glutathione-S-transfersase and, thus, is not a true microsomal mixed-function oxidase (see Section 1.3.6 on glutathione conjugation).

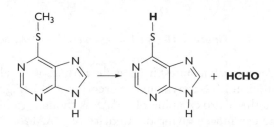

Figure 1.7 The S-demethylation of S-methylthiopurine.

(v)   *Oxidative deamination*. Amines containing the structure $-CH(CH_3)-NH_2$ are metabolised by the microsomal mixed-function oxidase system to release ammonium ions and leave the corresponding ketone. This is a different substrate specificity to the other enzyme metabolising amines, namely monoamine oxidase (MAO – see Section 1.2.2 (iv)) and the two enzymes do not

compete for the same substrates. Figure 1.8 shows the deamination of amphetamine. The ketone formed in this case is phenylmethylketone. As with
dealkylation, oxidative deamination involves an intermediate hydroxylation
step (Figure 1.9) with subsequent decomposition to yield the final products.

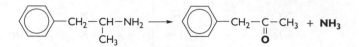

Figure 1.8 The oxidative deamination of amphetamine.

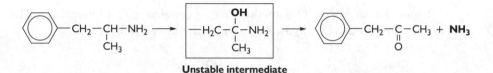

Unstable intermediate

Figure 1.9 The mechanism of oxidative deamination of amphetamine.

(vi)   *N-oxidation*. Hepatic microsomes in the presence of oxygen and NADPH
can form N-oxides. These oxidation products may be formed by the mixed-
function oxidase system or by separate flavoprotein N-oxidases. The enzyme
involved in N-oxidation depends on the substrate under study. Many different chemical groups can be N-oxidised including amines, amides, imines,
hydrazines and heterocyclic compounds. In Figure 1.10 the N-oxidation of
3-methylpyridine (a cytochrome P450-dependent reaction) is illustrated.

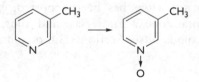

Figure 1.10 The N-oxidation of 3-methylpyridine.

N-oxidation may manifest itself as the formation of a hydroxylamine as in
the metabolism of 2-acetylaminofluorene (2-AAF) (Figure 1.11). This is of
interest as the hydroxylamine of 2-AAF is thought to be a precursor to the
proximate carcinogen giving the toxicity of 2-AAF.

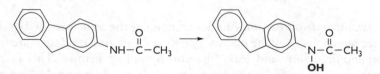

Figure 1.11 The N-hydroxylation of 2-acetylaminofluorene.

(vii) *S-oxidation.* Phenothiazines can be converted to their *S*-oxides (sulfoxides (S=O) and sulfones (=S=O)) by the microsomal mixed-function oxidase system. As an example the *S*-oxidation of chlorpromazine is shown in Figure 1.12.

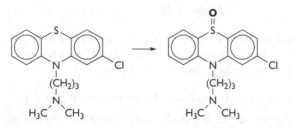

Figure 1.12 The S-oxidation of chlorpromazine.

(viii) *Phosphothionate oxidation.* The replacement of a phosphothionate sulfur atom with oxygen is a reaction common to the phosphothionate insecticides, e.g. parathion (Figure 1.13). The product paraoxon is a potent anticholinesterase and gives the potent insecticide action as well as the toxicity in humans.

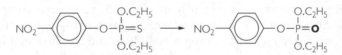

Figure 1.13 The oxidation of parathion.

(ix) *Dehalogenation.* The halogenated general anaesthetics, e.g. halothane, undergo oxidative dechlorination and debromination to yield the corresponding alcohol or acid (Figure 1.14).

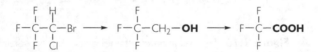

Figure 1.14 The oxidative dehalogenation of halothane.

One apparently unusual oxidation reaction performed by the mixed-function oxidase system is the conversion of ethanol to ethanal (acetaldehyde) (Figure 1.15). In this case the microsomal CYP2E1 appears to dehydrogenate ethanol as alcohol dehydrogenase does (see below). This may still be a hydroxylation reaction, however, as illustrated in Figure 1.15, but other mechanisms have also been proposed, including the formation of the hydroxyethyl radical.

The microsomal mixed-function oxidase system can, thus, catalyse a large range of oxidation reactions on a variety of substrates (Table 1.3). There is, however,

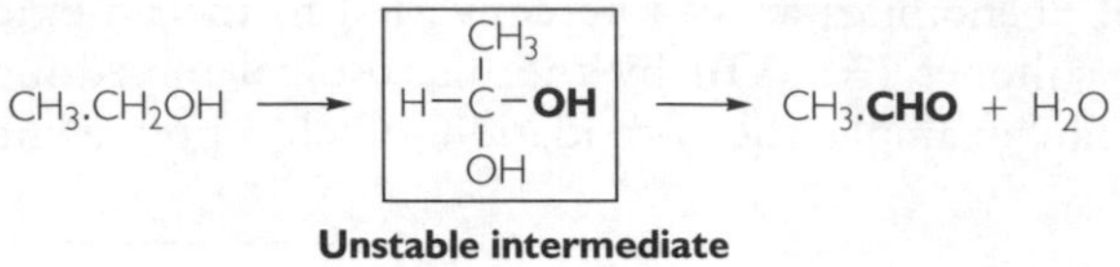

$$CH_3.CH_2OH \longrightarrow \boxed{\begin{array}{c} CH_3 \\ | \\ H-C-\textbf{OH} \\ | \\ OH \end{array}} \longrightarrow CH_3.\textbf{CHO} + H_2O$$

Unstable intermediate

Figure 1.15 The oxidation of ethanol.

another mixed-function oxidase system found in the mitochondria which is more selective in its substrates and is mainly involved in endogenous steroid metabolism (see Section 1.5 on endogenous metabolism).

1.2.2 Oxidations not catalysed by cytochrome P450

A number of enzymes in the body not related to cytochrome P450 can oxidise drugs. These are listed in Table 1.4.

Table 1.4 Oxidative enzymes other than mixed-function oxidases

Alcohol dehydrogenase
Aldehyde dehydrogenase
Xanthine oxidase
Amine oxidases
Aromatases
Alkylhydrazine oxidase

Most of these enzymes are primarily involved in endogenous compound metabolism and will be dealt with in the section related to that topic. A number, however, are more intimately involved in drug metabolism and are discussed below.

(i) *Alcohol dehydrogenase*. This enzyme catalyses the oxidation of many alcohols to the corresponding aldehyde and is localised in the soluble fraction of liver, kidney and lung cells. Unlike the CYP2E1 mentioned above, this enzyme uses NAD^+ as co-factor (Figure 1.16) and is a true dehydrogenase.

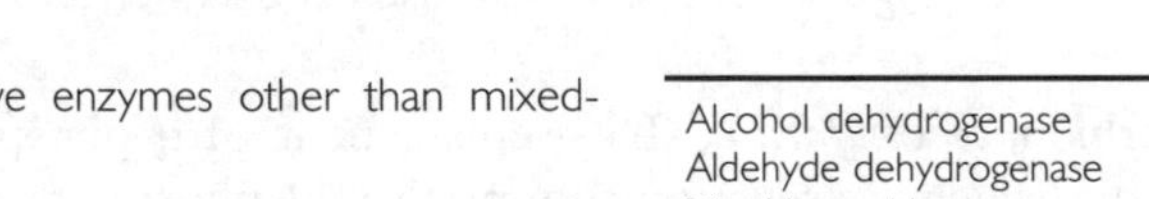

$$H_3C-\underset{\underset{H}{|}}{\overset{\overset{H}{|}}{C}}-OH + NAD^+ \longrightarrow H_3C-\overset{O}{\underset{H}{C}} + NADH + H^+$$

Figure 1.16 The oxidation of ethanol by alcohol dehydrogenase.

In naive animals the CYP2E1-mediated oxidation of ethanol is thought to be of minor importance but, following induction by ethanol, the microsomal oxidation of ethanol increases dramatically and may account for 80% of ethanol clearance in certain cases. In non-induced situations, alcohol dehydrogenase is the major metaboliser of ethanol.

(ii) *Aldehyde oxidation*. Aldehydes can be oxidised by a variety of enzymes involved in intermediary metabolism, e.g. aldehyde dehydrogenase, aldehyde oxidase and xanthine oxidase (the latter two being soluble metalloflavoproteins). The product of the reaction is the corresponding carboxylic acid (Figure 1.17).

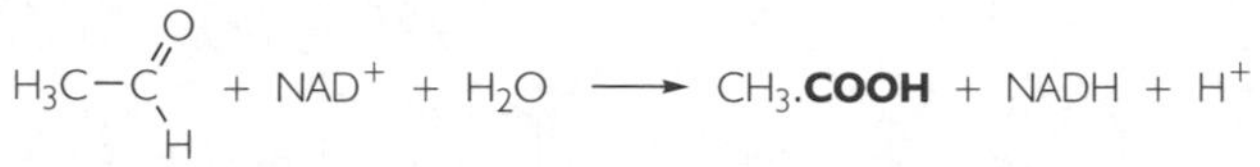

$$H_3C-\overset{\displaystyle O}{\underset{\displaystyle H}{C}} + NAD^+ + H_2O \longrightarrow CH_3.\textbf{COOH} + NADH + H^+$$

Figure 1.17 The oxidation of acetaldehyde.

(iii) *Xanthine oxidase.* This enzyme will metabolise xanthine-containing drugs, e.g. caffeine, theophylline and theobromine, and the purine analogues to the corresponding uric acid derivative (Figure 1.18).

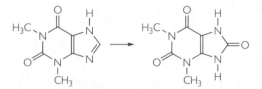

Figure 1.18 The oxidation of theophylline.

(iv) *Amine oxidases.* This group of enzymes can be subdivided into monoamine oxidases (responsible for the metabolism of endogenous catecholamines), diamine oxidases (deaminating endogenous diamines, e.g. histamine) and the flavoprotein *N*-oxidases and *N*-hydroxylases (which have been discussed above).

Monoamine oxidase metabolises dietary exogenous amines, e.g. tyramine (found in cheese, etc.) to the corresponding aldehyde (see Section 1.2.1(v)) and is found in mitochondria, at nerve endings and in the liver. The enzyme does not metabolise the amphetamine class of drugs that are metabolised by cytochrome P450.

Diamine oxidase is primarily involved with endogenous metabolism and is of little relevance here, whereas the *N*-oxidases are of importance in the metabolism of drugs, e.g. imipramine (Figure 1.19). These enzymes are found in liver microsomes. They appear to require NADPH and molecular oxygen, but are not mixed-function oxidases – they are flavoproteins.

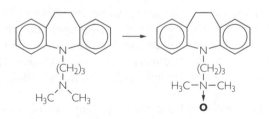

Figure 1.19 The *N*-oxidation of imipramine.

(v) *Aromatases.* Xenobiotics containing a cyclohexanecarboxylic acid group can be converted to the corresponding benzoic acid by a liver and kidney mitochondrial enzyme. The enzyme requires the co-enzyme A derivative of the acid as substrate, and oxygen and FAD as co-factors (Figure 1.20).

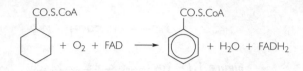

Figure 1.20 The aromatisation of cyclohexanecarboxylic acid CoA.

(vi) *Alkylhydrazine oxidase.* Carbidopa can be converted to 2-methyl-3',4'-di-hydroxyphenyl-propionic acid (Figure 1.21) by oxidation of the nitrogen function and subsequent rearrangement and decomposition of the inter-mediate. The exact mechanism is not known.

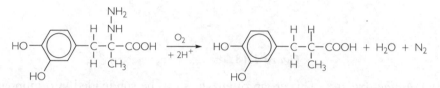

Figure 1.21 The oxidation of carbidopa.

1.2.3 Reductive metabolism

A number of reductive reactions can be catalysed by hepatic microsomal enzymes. These reactions usually require NADPH but are generally inhibited by oxygen, unlike the mixed-function oxidase reactions that require oxygen. A list of the types of compounds undergoing reduction is given in Table 1.5.

Table 1.5 Compounds undergoing reduction by hepatic microsomes

Azo-compounds
Nitro-compounds
Epoxides
Heterocyclic ring compounds
Halogenated hydrocarbons

Azo- and nitro-reduction can be catalysed by cytochrome P450 (but can also be catalysed by NADPH-cytochrome P450(c) reductase) and can involve substrates such as prontosil red (forming sulfanilamide) and chloramphenicol (Figure 1.22). The former reaction led to the discovery of the sulfonamides. The latter reaction is thought to occur in a stepwise fashion, as is seen in the reduction of nitrobenzene (Figure 1.23).

Epoxides can be converted back to the parent hydrocarbon, e.g. benzo(*a*)an-thracene-8,9-epoxide whereas some heterocyclic compounds can be ring cleaved by reduction (Figure 1.24). The products of the latter reaction are unstable and break down further to yield rearrangement and hydrolysis products.

Fluorocarbons of the halothane type can be defluorinated by liver microsomes in anaerobic conditions (cf. oxidative dehalogenation of halothane) as shown in Figure 1.25.

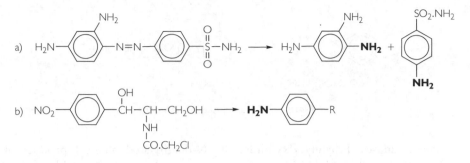

Figure 1.22 Reduction of (a) prontosil red and (b) chloramphenicol.

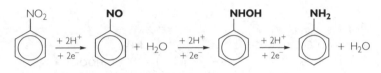

Figure 1.23 Stepwise reduction of aromatic nitro-group.

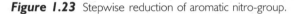

Figure 1.24 Ring cleavage of oxadiazoles.

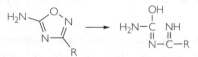

Figure 1.25 Reductive defluorination of halothane.

Steroid drugs with a Δ^4-double bond or a ring keto group can also be reduced by $5(\alpha/\beta)$ reductase and oxosteroid oxidoreductase, respectively.

1.2.4 Hydrolysis

Esters, amides, hydrazides and carbamates can readily be hydrolysed by various enzymes.

(i) *Ester hydrolysis.* The hydrolysis of esters can take place in the plasma (non-specific acetylcholinesterases, pseudocholinesterases and other esterases) or in the liver (specific esterases for particular groups of compounds). Procaine is metabolised by the plasma esterase (Figure 1.26) whereas pethidine (meperidine) is only metabolised by the liver esterase.

(ii) *Amide hydrolysis.* Amides may be hydrolysed by the plasma esterases (which are so non-specific that they will also hydrolyse amides, although more slowly than the corresponding esters) but are more likely to be hydrolysed by the

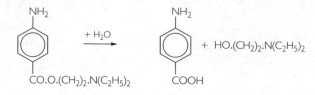

Figure 1.26 Hydrolysis of procaine.

liver amidases. Ethylglycylxylidide, the N-deethylated phase 1 product of lignocaine, is hydrolysed by the liver microsomal fraction to yield xylidine and ethylglycine (Figure 1.27).

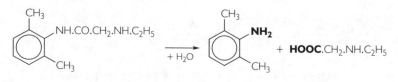

Figure 1.27 Hydrolysis of monoethylglycylxylidide.

(iii) *Hydrazide and carbamate hydrolysis.* Less common functional groups in drugs can also be hydrolysed, such as the hydrazide group in isoniazid (Figure 1.28) or the carbamate group in the previously used hypnotic, hedonal.

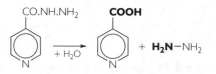

Figure 1.28 Hydrolysis of isoniazid.

The hydrolysis of proteins and peptides by enzymes can also be mentioned here but these enzymes are mainly found in gut secretions and are little involved in drug metabolism, except in the further metabolism of glutathione conjugates (see Section 1.3.6) and in the metabolism of peptide/protein drugs taken orally.

1.2.5 Hydration

Hydration can be regarded as a specialised form of hydrolysis where water is added to the compound without causing the compound to dissociate. Epoxides are particularly prone to hydration by the enzyme epoxide hydrolase, yielding the dihydrodiol. The precarcinogenic polycyclic hydrocarbon epoxides in particular undergo this reaction (e.g. benzo(a)pyrene-4,5-epoxide (Figure 1.29)). The reaction forms a *trans*-diol and, depending on the substrate, may be stereospecific.

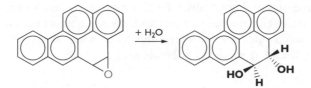

Figure 1.29 Hydration of benzo[a]pyrene-4,5-epoxide.

1.2.6 Other phase 1 reactions

Many other reactions which cannot be classified into the groups mentioned above have been proposed as possible routes of metabolism for specific drugs. A list of some of these reactions is given in Table 1.6. Further details of these reactions can be found in the reading list at the end of this chapter.

Table 1.6 Other reactions involved in drug metabolism

Reaction	Compound
Ring cyclisation	Proguanil
N-Carboxylation	Tocainide
Dimerisation	N-OH-2-Acetylaminofluorene
Transamidation	Propiram
Isomerisation	α-Methylfluorene-2-acetic acid
Decarboxylation	L-Dopa
Dethioacetylation	Spironolactone

1.2.7 Summary of phase 1 metabolism

As can be seen from the above, virtually every possible chemical reaction that a compound can undergo can be catalysed by the drug-metabolising enzyme systems. In most cases the final product contains a chemically reactive functional group, such as $-OH$, $-NH_2$, $-SH$, $-COOH$, etc., and, thus, as we shall see below, is in the correct chemical state to be acted upon by the phase 2 or conjugative enzymes. Indeed it is recognised that the main function of phase 1 metabolism is to prepare the compound for phase 2 metabolism and not to prepare the drug for excretion. Phase 2 is the true 'detoxication' of drugs and gives products that are generally water-soluble and easily excreted.

It will also be appreciated that many drugs can undergo a number of the reactions listed; indeed, some drugs can pass along many of the routes of metabolism described above. The importance of a particular pathway varies with many factors (most of which are described in Chapters 4 and 5) and it is obviously very difficult to predict the metabolism of a drug from the data given above. Computer-based expert systems for the prediction of routes of drug metabolism are available and are becoming more accurate as data is added to them but it is still not possible to fully predict the metabolism of a particular compound from its structure. Molecular graphical techniques, however, are giving a greater insight into the structure of the enzyme active sites and how substrates fit into the site. Such work should yield a model of substrate–enzyme interactions and, thus, a better understanding of the relationship between substrate structure and its metabolism. Further reading in this area will be found at the end of the chapter.

1.3 PHASE 2 METABOLISM

The phase 2 or conjugation reactions are listed in Table 1.7. It is seen that they involve a diverse group of enzymes often involving an 'activated' (or 'high-energy') co-factor or substrate derivative, generally leading to a water-soluble product which can be excreted in bile or urine.

Table 1.7 Conjugation reactions

Reaction	Enzyme	Functional group
Glucuronidation	UDP–Glucuronosyltransferase	$-OH$ $-COOH$ $-NH_2$ $-SH$
Glycosidation	UDP–Glycosyltransferase	$-OH$ $-COOH$ $-SH$
Sulfation	Sulfotransferase	$-NH_2$ $-SO_2NH_2$ $-OH$
Methylation	Methyltransferase	$-OH$ $-NH_2$
Acetylation	Acetyltransferase	$-NH_2$ $-SO_2NH_2$ $-OH$
Amino acid conjugation		$-COOH$
Glutathione conjugation	Glutathione-S-transferase	Epoxide Organic halide
Fatty acid conjugation		$-OH$
Condensation		Various

1.3.1 Conjugation with sugars

The major route of sugar conjugation is glucuronidation (conjugation with α-D-glucuronic acid) although conjugation with glucose, xylose and ribose are also possible, though, particularly in man, less common.

(i) *Glucuronidation.* Glucuronidation is the most widespread of the conjugation reactions probably due to the relative abundance of the co-factor for the reaction, UDP-glucuronic acid and the ubiquitous nature of the enzyme, UDP-glucuronosyltransferase. UDP-glucuronic acid, being part of the intermediary metabolism and closely related to glycogen synthesis, is found in all tissues

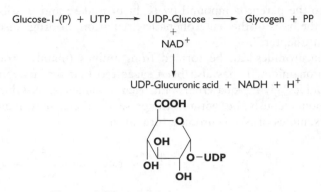

Glucose-1-(P) + UTP ⟶ UDP-Glucose ⟶ Glycogen + PP
+
NAD⁺
↓
UDP-Glucuronic acid + NADH + H⁺

Figure 1.30 Synthesis of UDP-glucuronic acid.

of the body (Figure 1.30). The enzymes involved are located in the cytosol. UDP-glucuronic acid can be considered as an energy-rich intermediate for the transfer of the glucuronic acid moiety.

Glucuronide formation is quantitatively the most important form of conjugation for drugs and endogenous compounds and can occur with alcohols, phenols, hydroxylamines, carboxylic acids, amines, sulfonamides and thiols.

O-Glucuronides form from phenols, alcohols and carboxylic acids – carboxylic acids forming 'ester' glucuronides and the others 'ether' glucuronides. Examples of each of these are shown in Figure 1.31. The reaction is the same in each case, requiring the microsomal enzyme, UDP-glucuronosyltransferase. It is interesting to note that inversion takes place during the reaction with the α-glucuronic acid forming a β-glucuronide. The O-glucuronides are often excreted in bile and thus released into the gut where they can be broken

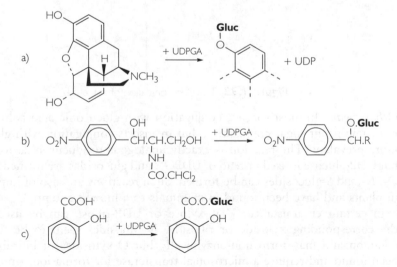

Figure 1.31 The glucuronidation of (a) morphine, (b) chloramphenicol and (c) salicylic acid.

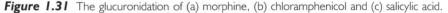

down to the parent compound by β-glucuronidase and possibly reabsorbed. This is the basis of the 'enterohepatic circulation' of drugs discussed in more detail in Chapter 7.

N-Glucuronides can be formed from amines (mainly aromatic), amides and sulfonamides. It has also been suggested that tertiary amines can form glucuronides giving quaternary nitrogen conjugates. N-Glucuronides may form spontaneously, i.e. without the presence of enzymes. Figure 1.32 shows some examples of N-glucuronide formation.

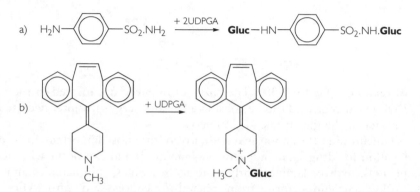

Figure 1.32 The glucuronidation of (a) sulfanilamide and (b) cyproheptidine.

Thiol groups can react with UDPGA in the presence of UDP-glucuronosyl-transferase to yield S-glucuronides. An example of this is given in Figure 1.33 with antabuse as substrate.

Direct attachment of glucuronic acid to the carbon skeleton of drugs has also been reported (i.e. C-glucuronidation).

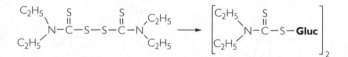

Figure 1.33 The glucuronidation of antabuse.

(ii) *Other sugars*. In most species, conjugation with glucuronic acid is by far the most important sugar conjugation, but in insects conjugation with glucose is more prevalent. The reaction is exactly analogous to glucuronide formation but UDP-glucose is used instead of UDPGA and glucosides are formed. Similar O-, N- and S-glucosides can be formed. Such reactions are also of importance in plants and have been found in mammals to a limited extent.

In certain circumstances UDP-xylose or UDP-ribose can be used giving the corresponding xyloside or riboside. N-Ribosides seem to be the most common and may form non-enzymically but O-xylosides of bilirubin have been found and require a microsomal transferase for formation. An example of an N-riboside formation is shown in Figure 1.34.

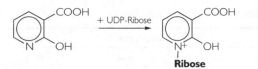

Figure 1.34 The *N*-ribosylation of 2-hydroxynicotinic acid.

1.3.2 Sulfation

Sulfation is a major conjugation pathway for phenols but can also occur for alcohols, amines and, to a lesser extent, thiols. As with sugar conjugation, an energy-rich donor is required – in this case 3'-phosphoadenosine-5'-phosphosulfate (PAPS) (Figure 1.35). PAPS is produced by a two-stage reaction from ATP and sulfate as illustrated in Figure 1.36. These reactions occur in the cytosol.

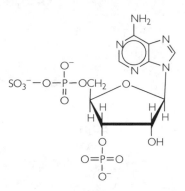

Figure 1.35 The structure of PAPS.

$$SO_4^{2-} + ATP \xrightarrow{\text{ATP-sulfurylase}} \text{Adenosine-5'-phosphosulfate (APS)} + PP_i$$

$$APS + ATP \xrightarrow{\text{APS-kinase}} \text{3'-Phosphoadenosine-5'-phosphosulfate (PAPS)} + ADP$$

Figure 1.36 The formation of PAPS.

Sulfation occurs by interaction of the drug and PAPS in the presence of the cytosolic enzyme, sulfotransferase. Various forms of the enzyme have been described named after their preferred substrates although classification by molecular and gene structure is becoming more common (see Chapter 2) – a list of these is given in Table 1.8.

The phenol, alcohol and arylamine sulfotransferases are fairly non-specific and will metabolise a wide range of drugs and xenobiotics but the steroid sulfotransferases are specific for a single steroid or a number of steroids of a particular type. For example, oestrone sulfotransferase will sulfate oestrone and, to a lesser extent, other estrogens while testosterone is sulfated by another sulfotransferase. Some examples of sulfate conjugation are shown in Figure 1.37.

Table 1.8 Sulfotransferases and their substrates

Isoenzyme	Substrate	Site
Phenol sulfotransferase	Isoprenaline	Liver
		Kidney
		Gut
Alcohol sulfotransferase	Dimetranidazole	Liver
Steroid sulfotransferase	Oestrone	Liver
Arylamine sulfotransferase	Paracetamol	Liver

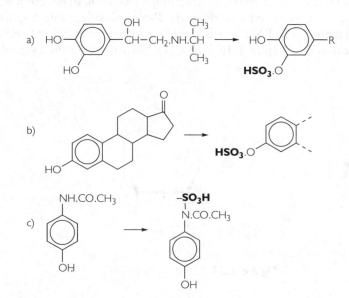

Figure 1.37 Sulfate conjugation of (a) isoprenaline, (b) oestrone and (c) paracetamol.

As is seen, most drugs and endogenous compounds that can be glucuronidated can also be sulfated and this leads to the possibility of competition for the substrate between the two pathways. In general sulfate conjugation predominates at low substrate concentration and glucuronide conjugation at high concentration due to the kinetics of the two reactions and the limited supply of PAPS in the cell compared to UDPGA.

1.3.3 Methylation

Methylation reactions are mainly involved with endogenous compound metabolism but some drugs may be methylated by non-specific methyltransferases found in lung, and by the physiological methyltransferases. A list of the methyltransferases and their substrates is given in Table 1.9.

The co-factor, *S*-adenosylmethionine (SAM), is required to form methyl conjugates and is produced from L-methionine and ATP under the influence of

Table 1.9 The methyltransferases

Enzyme	Substrate	Site
Phenylethanolamine N-methyltransferase	Noradrenaline	Adrenals
Non-specific N-methyltransferase	Various (desmethylimipramine)	Lung
Imidazole N-methyltransferase	Histamine	Liver
Catechol O-methyltransferase	Catechols	Liver Kidney Skin Nerve tissue
Hydroxyindole O-methyltransferase	N-Acetylserotonin	Pineal gland
S-Methyltransferase	Thiols	Liver Kidney Lung

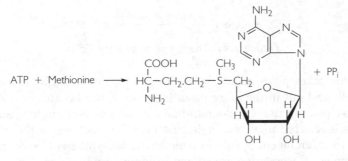

Figure 1.38 The formation of S-adenosylmethionine.

the enzyme, L-methionine adenosyltransferase (Figure 1.38). SAM can also be considered as a high-energy intermediate (cf. UDPGA and PAPS above).

The non-specific N-methyltransferase found in the lung can reverse the N-demethylation reactions of phase 1 metabolism (see Figure 1.39) but most of the other methyltransferases are specific for endogenous compounds (see Section 1.5 on endogenous metabolism) except the S-methyltransferase that is found in the microsomal fraction and which will methylate many thiols (see Figure 1.40) such as thiouracil.

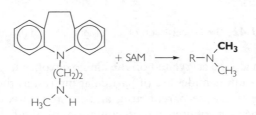

Figure 1.39 The N-methylation of desmethylimipramine.

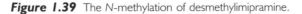

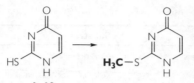

Figure 1.40 The S-methylation of thiouracil.

In general, unlike other conjugation reactions, methylation leads to a less polar product and thus hinders excretion of the drug.

1.3.4 Acetylation

Acetylation reactions are common for aromatic amines and sulfonamides and require the co-factor, acetyl-CoA, which may be obtained from the glycolysis pathway or via direct interaction of acetate and coenzyme A (Figure 1.41).

$$CH_3.COO^- + CoASH \xrightarrow{\text{CoA-S-acetyltransferase}} CH_3.CO.S.CoA$$

Figure 1.41 The formation of acetyl-CoA.

Acetylation takes place mainly in the liver and, interestingly, is found in the Kupffer cells and not in the more usual location of the hepatocytes. Acetylation can also take place in the reticuloendothelial cells of the spleen, lung and gut, and the enzyme is referred to as N-acetyltransferase. The location of the enzyme may be related to its endogenous role in leukotriene biosynthesis (see Section 1.5.2). Some examples of acetylation are shown in Figure 1.42.

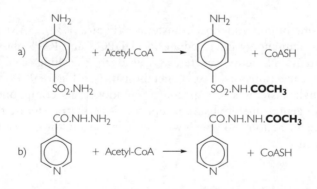

Figure 1.42 The N-acetylation of (a) sulfanilamide and (b) isoniazid.

Sulfanilamide can also be acetylated on the amine nitrogen to give a diacetylated product. The acetyl-sulfonamides are of particular interest as they are appreciably less soluble in water than the parent drug and the renal toxicity of the earlier sulfonamides has been attributed to precipitation of these conjugates in the kidney.

1.3.5 Amino acid conjugation

Exogenous carboxylic acids, in common with acetate noted above, can form CoA derivatives in the body under the action of the enzyme, ATP-dependent acid: CoA ligase, and can then react with endogenous amines, such as amino acids, to form conjugates. Amino acid conjugation is, thus, a special form of N-acylation, where the drug and not the endogenous co-factor is activated. The usual amino acids involved are glycine, glutamine, ornithine, arginine and taurine. The generalised reaction is given in Figure 1.43. This pathway was implicated in the first described production of a drug metabolite by Keller in 1842 when hippuric acid was found as a urinary excretion product of benzoic acid (Figure 1.44).

$$R-COOH + ATP \longrightarrow R-CO-AMP + PPi$$
$$R-CO-AMP + CoASH \longrightarrow R-CO.S.CoA + AMP$$
$$R-CO.S.CoA + R'-NH_2 \longrightarrow R-CO.NH-R' + CoASH$$

Figure 1.43 The amino acid conjugation of carboxylic acids.

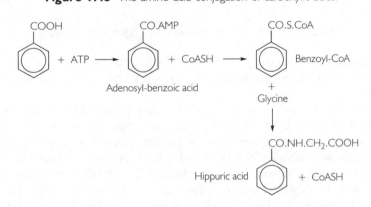

Figure 1.44 The glycine conjugation of benzoic acid.

The particular amino acid used is related to the intermediary metabolism of the species under study such that ureotelic animals (those excreting urea) tend to use glycine while uricotelic species (those excreting uric acid) use predominantly ornithine.

1.3.6 Glutathione conjugation

Glutathione is recognised as a protective compound within the body for the removal of potentially toxic electrophilic compounds. Many drugs either are, or can be, metabolised by phase 1 reactions to strong electrophiles, and these can react with glutathione to form (in general) non-toxic conjugates. The list of compounds conjugated to glutathione includes epoxides, haloalkanes, nitroalkanes, alkenes, and aromatic halo- and nitro-compounds. Examples of these are given in Figure 1.45. The enzymes catalysing the above reactions are the glutathione-S-transferases which are located in the cytosol of liver, kidney, gut and other tissues.

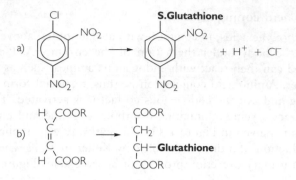

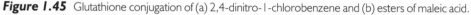

Figure 1.45 Glutathione conjugation of (a) 2,4-dinitro-1-chlorobenzene and (b) esters of maleic acid.

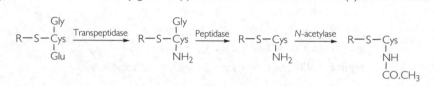

Figure 1.46 The further metabolism of a glutathione conjugate.

The glutathione conjugates may be excreted directly in urine, or more usually bile, but more often further metabolism of the conjugate takes place, as illustrated in Figure 1.46.

The tripeptide glutathione (Gly–Cys–Glu), once attached to the acceptor molecule, can be attacked by a γ-glutamyltranspeptidase, which removes the glutamate, and a peptidase, which removes the glycine, to yield the cysteine conjugate. These enzymes are found in the liver and kidney cytosol. N-Acetylation of the cysteine conjugate can then occur via the normal N-acetylation pathway described above to yield the N-acetylcysteine conjugate or mercapturic acid. The glycylcysteine and cysteine conjugates and the mercapturic acids are all found as

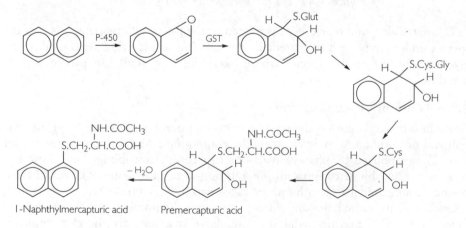

Figure 1.47 The phase 1 and 2 metabolism of naphthalene.

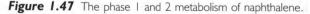

excretion products, depending on the substrate and species under study. One example of this complete process is found for the metabolism of naphthalene (Figure 1.47).

As well as being broken down by this process, sulfur-containing conjugates secreted in bile can also be further metabolised by an enzyme in the gut called C–S lyase or cysteine conjugate β-lyase. This idea has been further expanded when dealing with certain sulfur-containing compounds or compounds that form sulfur-containing conjugates, such as 2-acetamido-4(chloromethyl)-thiazole, caffeine and propachlor. In these cases the methylthio-derivates found as excretion products have been postulated to arise as shown in Figure 1.48. The breakdown of the glutathione conjugate is performed by a C–S lyase in the intestinal microflora transferring the −SH group from glutathione to the substrate, where subsequent S-methylation and reabsorption take place. The S-methylated compound is oxidised in the liver to a methylthio-derivative and then excreted. The series of reactions for the anti-inflammatory drug, 2-acetamido-4-chloromethyl-thiazole is shown in Figure 1.49.

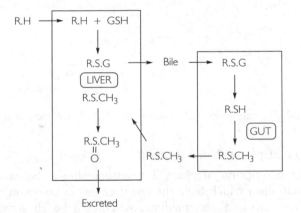

Figure 1.48 Phase 3 metabolism.

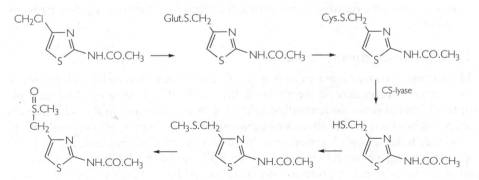

Figure 1.49 The metabolism of 2-acetamido-4-chloromethylthiazole.

The glutathione transferases have also been implicated in the denitrosation reaction of a range of substrates (e.g. glyceryl trinitrate – an anti-anginal compound and explosive). The potential release of nitric oxide (NO) during this reaction is of great significance as NO is known to be a powerful endogenous signalling molecule involved in regulation of smooth muscle tone in, for example, blood vessels. This is thought to be how glyceryl trinitrate gives its anti-anginal effects.

1.3.7 Fatty acid conjugation

Fatty acid conjugation has been shown to occur for 11-hydroxy-9-tetrahydro-cannabinol (the active ingredient in cannabis resin). The fatty acids involved are stearic and palmitic acid (Figure 1.50). The microsomal fraction from liver catalyses this reaction. Little is known, however, of the mechanism or whether other compounds can be conjugated in this way.

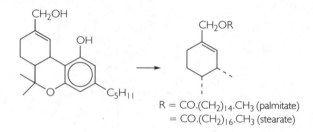

$R = CO.(CH_2)_{14}.CH_3$ (palmitate)
$ = CO.(CH_2)_{16}.CH_3$ (stearate)

Figure 1.50 The conjugation of 11-hydroxy-Δ^9-THC to palmitic and stearic acids.

1.3.8 Summary of phase 2 metabolism

The above brief description of phase 2 reactions shows the range of possible products of metabolism which have the requirement in common for some form of energy-rich or 'activated' intermediate, whether it be an activated co-factor (e.g. UDPGA, PAPS, SAM, acetyl coenzyme A) or an activated drug. In the main, phase 2 metabolites are more water-soluble (cf. N-methylation) and conjugation reactions are regarded as preparing the drug for excretion by one pathway or another.

1.3.9 Stereoselective reactions

Many drugs in common use are optically active and it has become clear that some of the optical isomers may be metabolised differently. The best researched example of this is probably the anticoagulant, warfarin. Warfarin exists in R- and S-isomers and the S-isomer is metabolised more rapidly than the R-isomer. This generalisation, however, hides a complex stereospecific and regiospecific metabolism, with the R-isomer being extensively metabolised by CYP3A4 to the 10-hydroxy derivative whereas the S-isomer is preferentially metabolised by CYP2C9 to 7-hydroxywarfarin (CYP3A4 appears to produce dehydrowarfarin from the S-isomer).

1.4 SUMMARY OF DRUG-METABOLISING REACTIONS

In the preceding pages the various reactions that drugs can undergo have been described and the relative importance of the reactions discussed. It will be seen that very many different reactions can be found, depending on the drug under study. A book of this type cannot hope to cover all of these reactions but it is hoped, however, that this chapter has given some insight into the complexity of drug metabolism and the interactions of the complementary, sequential and competing pathways. It should be possible by using the information given above to work out how a drug *may* be metabolised.

The final section of this chapter deals with the interrelationship of drug and endogenous compound metabolism in an attempt to indicate where the overlap between the two may occur and how this may lead to interactions.

1.5 ENDOGENOUS METABOLISM RELATED TO DRUG METABOLISM

The enzymes discussed above, the 'drug-metabolising' enzymes, are a diverse group performing a range of different reactions. As well as biotransforming many drugs, the majority of the enzymes also metabolise endogenous compounds and it has been suggested that the true function of these enzymes is in endogenous metabolism, so it is purely fortuitous that they also metabolise drugs and other xenobiotics. The greater affinity for the 'natural' substrate in many cases would seem to support this idea but this evidence is not conclusive. Some of the enzymes shown above are also thought to be protective – detoxifying potentially harmful chemicals in the environment – and, thus, have little role to play in endogenous metabolism. It is, however, accepted that the same enzymes metabolise exogenous and endogenous compounds in many cases.

In this section we will look at endogenous metabolism catalysed by the 'drug-metabolising' enzymes discussed above.

1.5.1 Phase 1

(i) *Mixed-function oxidase.* Phase 1 metabolism is dominated by the mixed-function oxidase system (cytochrome P450) and this is known to be involved in the metabolism of steroid hormones, thyroid hormones, fatty acids, prostaglandins and derivatives.

The metabolism of steroids is intimately linked to that of drugs, as can be seen from the common developmental patterns and physiological control (see Chapter 4). Indeed, steroid biosynthesis is dependent on cytochrome P450 at many stages. This may be of the microsomal or mitochondrial type of mixed-function oxidase (see Chapter 2), depending on the reaction being studied. The importance of this enzyme is best illustrated by looking at the biosynthesis of steroids from cholesterol.

The rate-limiting step in steroid biosynthesis is the conversion of cholesterol to pregnenolone and this is a multi-stage reaction referred to as side-chain

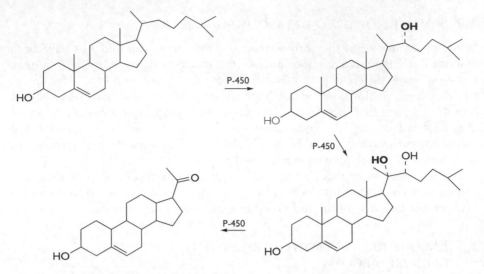

Figure 1.51 The conversion of cholesterol to pregnenolone.

cleavage (Figure 1.51). A specific form of cytochrome P450 has been isolated from the mitochondria of steroid-producing tissues that perform the above reaction. It is seen that the first two steps are simple aliphatic hydroxylations and require NADPH and molecular oxygen as co-factors (cf. drug metabolism).

The further metabolism of pregnenolone also involves the mixed-function oxidase at many stages (Figure 1.52), some of which take place in the microsomal fraction and some in the mitochondria. Most of the reactions are found predominantly in the steroid-synthesising tissues but may also be seen elsewhere.

Thus we have cholesterol side-chain cleavage, 11β-, 17α- and 21-hydroxylations and aromatisation of androgens all dependent on cytochrome P450.

The breakdown of steroids by the liver and other tissues is also, to a great extent, dependent on the mixed-function oxidase system. All steroids are hydroxylated in various positions by this enzyme system and, in most cases, the metabolites are less active. One such example is androst-4-ene-3,17-dione (the precursor of the male sex hormone, testosterone) which is hydroxylated at the 6β-, 7α- and 16α- positions preferentially (Figure 1.53). The enzymes in this case are located in the microsomal fraction of the liver and are exactly the same enzymes that metabolise drugs. Other steroids are hydroxylated in different positions by the same enzymes.

A somewhat different scheme is seen for vitamin D (Figure 1.54). After ring opening by UV light of 7-dehydrocholesterol to yield vitamin D$_3$, the vitamin is converted to its active form by 25-hydroxylation in the liver and subsequent 1-hydroxylation by the kidney mitochondria. Both of the hydroxylations are catalysed by mixed-function oxidases.

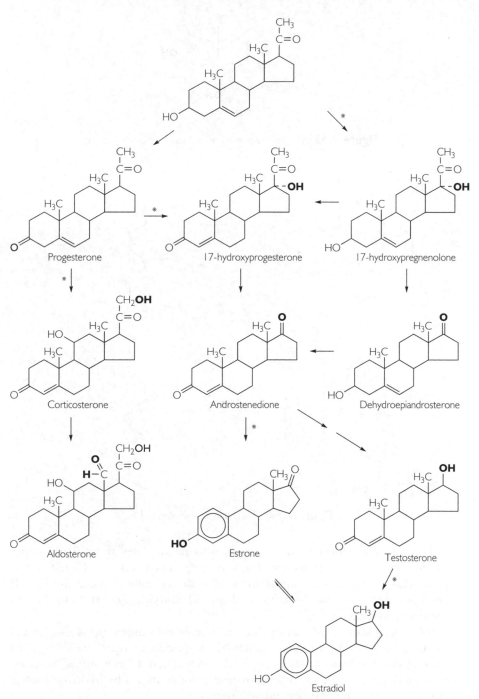

Figure 1.52 The biosynthesis of steroid hormones from pregnenolone. * = cytochrome P450-dependent.

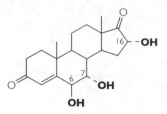

Figure 1.53 The hydroxylation of androst-4-ene-3,17-dione.

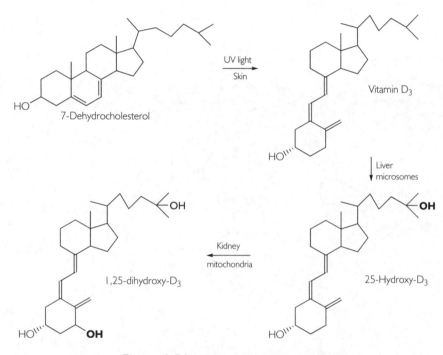

Figure 1.54 The activation of vitamin D_3.

The mixed-function oxidase system also metabolises thyroid hormones by de-iodination (a mechanism for saving the body's store of iodine) and fatty acids. Fatty acids are metabolised by hydroxylation in the ω and $(\omega - 1)$ positions and can also be converted to the epoxide and thus to the di-hydroxyacid (Figure 1.55).

It has been postulated that the biosynthesis of prostaglandins is also related to the mixed-function oxidase system in requiring cytochrome P450. The prostaglandin synthetase enzyme is closely related to the mixed-function oxidase (Figure 1.56). The breakdown of prostaglandins by hydroxylation is also a cytochrome P450-dependent process.

(ii) *Other oxidations.* Other oxidation reactions, which are not cytochrome P450-dependent but are related to drug metabolism, occur with endogenous

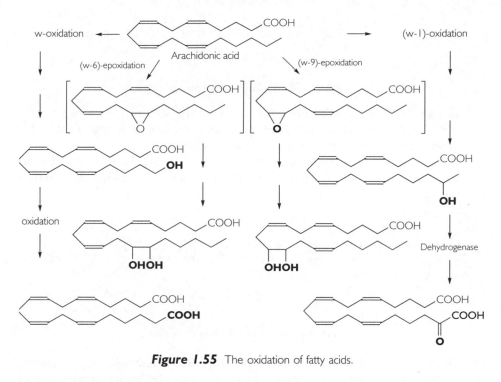

Figure 1.55 The oxidation of fatty acids.

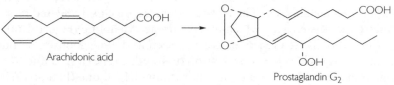

Figure 1.56 The prostaglandin synthetase reaction.

compounds. The oxosteroid oxidoreductases, for instance, are able to oxidise alcohols to ketones but their physiological function is in steroid metabolism (Figure 1.57).

The monoamine oxidase is primarily an enzyme to break down endogenous neurotransmitters, e.g. norepinephrine (noradrenaline) (Figure 1.58), but it

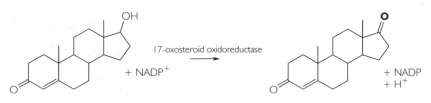
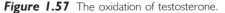

Figure 1.57 The oxidation of testosterone.

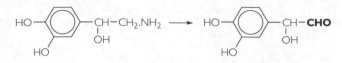

Figure 1.58 The oxidation of norepinephrine.

can also metabolise exogenous amines of similar structure (cf. drug metabolism, earlier in this chapter) whereas diamine oxidase deaminates the endogenous amines, histamine, putrescine and cadaverine.

The xanthine oxidases are primarily related to breakdown of endogenous purines to uric acid via xanthine (Figure 1.59) for subsequent excretion
in urine.

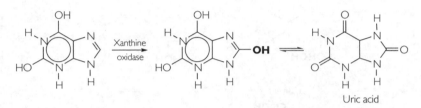

Figure 1.59 The oxidation of xanthine.

(iii) *Other phase 1 reactions.* Of the other phase 1 reactions noted above,
hydrolysis is the one which shows the most overlap between endogenous and
exogenous metabolism. The plasma esterases are closely related to acetylcho-
linesterase, the enzyme which inactivates acetylcholine (Figure 1.60).

Certain reduction reactions are also seen in the metabolism of endogenous
compounds such as the conversation of 4-androstene-3,17-dione to testosterone (see Figure 1.52) and to 5α-androstane-3,17-dione (Figure 1.61) but the
relationship of these reactions to the reduction of drug substrates is unclear.

A summary of phase 1 reactions related to endogenous metabolism is given in
Table 1.10.

$$CH_3.CO.O.CH_2.CH_2.\overset{+}{N}(CH_3)_3 \longrightarrow CH_3.COO^- + HO.CH_2.CH_2.\overset{+}{N}(CH_3)_3$$

acetate   choline

Figure 1.60 The hydrolysis of acetylcholine.

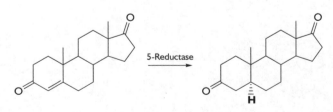

Figure 1.61 The 5α-reduction of androst-4-ene-3,17-dione.

Table 1.10 Endogenous metabolism by phase I enzymes

Enzyme	Endogenous substrates
Mixed-function oxidase	Steroids
	Sterols
	Thyroid hormones
	Fatty acids
	Prostaglandins
	Vitamin D
	Leukotrienes
Monoamine oxidase	Monoamine neurotransmitters
Diamine oxidase	Histamine
	Putrescine
	Cadaverine
Xanthine oxidase	Xanthine
Hydroxysteroid oxidoreductase	Steroids
Acetylcholinesterase	Acetylcholine
Reductases	Steroids

1.5.2 Phase 2

(i) *Glucuronidation.* Glucuronidation is a common pathway of metabolism for many endogenous compounds including steroid hormones, catecholamines, bilirubin and thyroxine. As with glucuronidation of drugs, this process is a preparation for excretion of the compound. Many steroids are excreted as glucuronides into the bile and thus in the faeces. The excretion of bilirubin is dependent on glucuronide formation, and the liver contains a specific form of UDP-glucuronosyltransferase for bilirubin. An example of steroid glucuronide formation is shown in Figure 1.62.

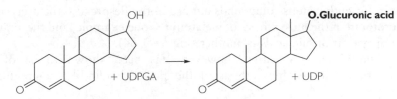

Figure 1.62 The formation of testosterone 17-glucuronide.

(ii) *Sulfation.* Sulfate formation is involved in the biosynthesis of steroids and heparin, each of which have specific sulfotransferases and do not interfere to any great extent with drug metabolism.

(iii) *Methylation.* Methylation is predominantly a reaction involving endogenous compounds, although certain exogenous compounds may also be metabolised (see above). The methyltransferases are listed in Table 1.9 and include phenylethanolamine *N*-methyltransferase (PNMT) that converts norepinephrine (noradrenaline) to epinephrine (adrenaline) in the adrenal gland, imidazole

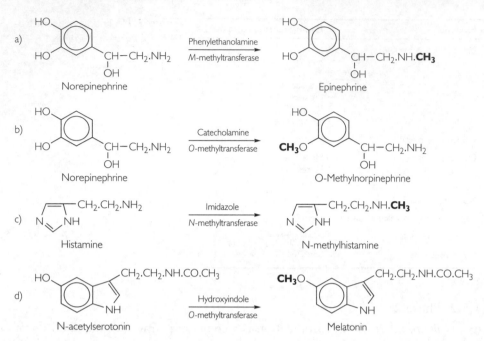

Figure 1.63 Examples of endogenous methyltransferases.

N-methyltransferase (IMT) which inactivates histamine in the liver, catechol O-methyltransferase (COMT) which inactivates catecholamines mainly in nerve cells and liver, and hydroxy-indole-O-methyltransferase (HIOMT) which synthesises melatonin in the pineal gland (Figure 1.63).

(iv) *Other phase 2 reactions.* Acetylation and amino acid conjugation reactions are seen for endogenous compounds but are not widespread – the acetylation of serotonin in the biosynthesis of melatonin is one example, and the amino acid conjugation of bile acids is another (Figure 1.64).

Glutathione conjugation, however, has been shown to be of major importance in the biosynthesis of the prostaglandin-like compounds, the

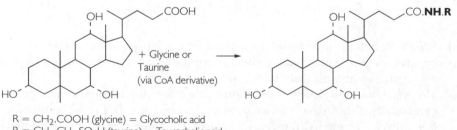

R = CH$_2$.COOH (glycine) = Glycocholic acid
R = CH$_2$.CH$_2$.SO$_3$H (taurine) = Taurocholic acid

Figure 1.64 The amino acid conjugation of bile acids.

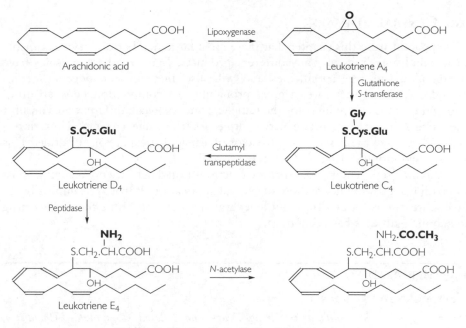

Figure 1.65 The biosynthesis of the leukotrienes.

leukotrienes. In fact, leukotriene synthesis involves phase 1 and 2 metabolism and is very similar to the metabolism of naphthalene (see Figure 1.47) involving epoxide formation, glutathione conjugation and breakdown of the conjugate to yield, finally, the cysteine conjugate and the mercapturic acid (Figure 1.65).

A summary of phase 2 reactions involving endogenous compounds is given in Table 1.11.

Table 1.11 Phase 2 metabolism of endogenous compounds

Reaction	Substrates
Glucuronidation	Steroids
	Thyroxine
	Bilirubin
	Catecholamines
Sulfation	Steroids
	Carbohydrates
Methylation	Biogenic amines
Acetylation	Serotonin
Amino acid conjugation	Bile acids
Glutathione conjugation	Arachidonic acid metabolites (leukotrienes)

1.6 GENERAL SUMMARY

It is apparent from this chapter that there are a large number of enzymes capable of metabolising drugs to many different products. Many of these enzymes have overlapping substrate specificities and will also metabolise endogenous compounds. There is, therefore, a great probability of competition between drugs and endogenous compounds for the same enzyme, between different enzymes for the same substrate and between two drugs for the same enzyme. These interactions are often the basis for the toxic or pharmacological actions of drugs. This is discussed in more detail in Chapters 6 and 7.

It should also be emphasised that the reactions noted here are not a complete list of possible reactions but are those of general application. It would be impossible to give all reactions for all drugs, but a general appreciation of the most likely drug metabolic pathways has been given.

FURTHER READING

Textbooks and symposia

Damani, L.A. (1989) *Sulphur-containing Drugs and Related Compounds: Chemistry, Biochemistry and Toxicology*. Vols 1 & 2, Ellis Horwood, Chichester.

Fishman, W.H. (1961) *Chemistry of Drug Metabolism*. Thomas, Springfield.

Hawkins, D.R. (1988–1996) *Biotransformations: A Survey of the Biotransformations of Drugs and Chemicals in Animals*. Vols 1–7, Royal Society of Chemistry, London.

Ioannides, C. (1996) *Cytochromes P450: Metabolic and Toxicological Aspects*. CRC Press, Boca Raton, FL.

Mulder, G.J. (ed.) (1990) *Conjugation Reactions in Drug Metabolism*. Taylor & Francis, London.

Parke, D.V. (1968) *The Biochemistry of Foreign Compounds*. Pergamon, Oxford.

Testa, B. (1995) *The Metabolism of Drugs and Other Xenobiotics: Biochemistry of Redox Reactions*. Academic Press, London.

Williams, R.T. (1959) *Detoxification Mechanisms*. Chapman and Hall, London.

Woolf, T.F. (ed.) (1999) *Handbook of Drug Metabolism*. Marcel Dekker, New York.

Reviews and original articles

Albano, E. *et al.* (1991) Role of ethanol-inducible cytochrome P450 (P4502E1) in catalysing the free radical activation of aliphatic alcohols. *Biochem. Pharmacol.* **41**, 1895–1902.

Anders, M.W. and Dekant, M.W. (1998) Glutathione-dependent bioactivation of haloalkenes. *Ann. Rev. Pharmacol. Toxicol.* **38**, 501–537.

Beedham, C. (1997) The role of non-P450 enzymes in drug oxidation. *Pharm. World Sci.* **19**, 255–263.

Capdevila, J.H. *et al.* (1992) Cytochrome P450 and the arachidonate cascade. *FASEB J.* **6**, 731–736.

Gasser, R. (1996) The flavin-containing monooxygenase system. *Exp. Toxicol. Pathol.* **48**, 467–470.

George, J. and Farrell, G.C. (1991) Role of human hepatic cytochromes P450 in drug metabolism and toxicity. *Aust. NZ J. Med.* **21**, 356–362.

Gonzalez, F.J. and Nebert, D.W. (1990) Evolution of the P450 gene superfamily. *TIG* **6**, 182–186.

Guengerich, F.P. (1992) Human cytochrome P450 enzymes. *Life Sci.* **50**, 1471–1478.

Halkier, B.A. (1996) Catalytic reactivities and structure/function relationships of cytochrome P450 enzymes. *Phytochemistry* **43**, 1–21.

Hawes, E.M. (1998) N^+-Glucuronidation: a common pathway in human metabolism of drugs with a tertiary amine group. *Drug Metab. Disp.* **26**, 830–837.

Honkakoski, P. and Negishi, M. (1997) The structure, function and regulation of cytochrome P450 2A enzymes. *Drug Metab. Rev.* **29**, 977–996.

Ingelman-Sundberg, M. *et al.* (1990) Drug metabolizing enzymes: genetics, regulation and toxicology. *Proceedings of the VIIIth International Symposium on Microsomes and Drug Oxidations, Stockholm.*

Jensen, D.E. *et al.* (1997) Denitrosation of 1,3-dimethyl-2-cyano-1-nitrosoguanidine in rat primary hepatocyte cultures. *Biochem. Pharmacol.* **53**, 1297–1306.

Kaminsky, L.S. and Zhang, Z.-Y. (1996) Human P450 metabolism of warfarin. *Pharmacol. Ther.* **73**, 67–74.

Knights, K.M. (1998) Role of hepatic fatty acid:coenzyme A ligases in the metabolism of xenobiotic carboxylic acids. *Clin. Exp. Pharmacol. Physiol.* **25**, 776–782.

Koop, D.R. (1992) Oxidative and reductive metabolism by cytochrome P450 2E1. *FASEB J.* **6**, 724–730.

Kroemer, H.K. and Klotz, U. (1992) Glucuronidation of drugs. *Clin. Pharmacokin.* **23**, 292–310.

Kumar, R. (1984) Metabolism of 1,25-dihydroxy vitamin D_3. *Physiol. Rev.* **64**, 478–504.

Larsen, G.L. *et al.* (1988) *In vitro* metabolism of the methylthio group of 2-methyl-thiobenzothiazole by rat liver. *Xenobiotica* **18**, 313–322.

Lewis, D.F.V. (1998) The CYP2 family: Models, mutants and interactions. *Xenobiotica* **28**, 617–661.

Lewis, D.F.V. *et al.* (1998) Structural determinants of cytochrome P450 substrate specificity, binding affinity and catalytic rate. *Chemico-Biol. Interact.* **115**, 175–199.

Niwa, T. *et al.* (1998) Contribution of human hepatic cytochrome P450 isoforms to regioselective hydroxylation of steroid hormones. *Xenobiotica* **28**, 539–547.

Rendic, S. and Di Carlo, F.J. (1997) Human cytochrome P450 enzymes: a status report summarizing their reactions, substrates, inducers and inhibitors. *Drug Metab. Rev.* **29**, 413–580.

Segall, M.D. *et al.* (1997) *Ab initio* molecular modelling in the study of drug metabolism. *Eur. J. Drug Metab. Pharmacokin.* **22**, 283–289.

Smith, D.A. *et al.* (1997) Properties of cytochrome P450 isoenzymes and their substrates. *Drug Disc. Today* **2**, 406–414.

Smith, G. *et al.* (1998) Molecular genetics of the human cytochrome P450 monooxygenase superfamily. *Xenobiotica* **28**, 1129–1165.

Soucek, P. and Gut, I. (1992) Cytochromes P450 in rats. Structures, functions, properties and relevant human forms. *Xenobiotica* **22**, 83–103.

Takemori, S. and Kominami, S. (1984) The role of cytochrome P450 in adrenal steroidogenesis. *TIPS* **9**, 393–396.

Tephly, T.R. and Burchell, B. (1990) UDP-glucuronosyltransferases, a family of detoxifying enzymes. *TIPS* **11**, 276–279.

Tracy, T.S. (1995) Stereochemistry in pharmacotherapy: when mirror images are not identical. *Ann. Pharmacother.* **29**, 161–165.

Waxman, D.J. (1988) Interactions of hepatic cytochrome P450 with steroid hormones. *Biochem. Pharmacol.* **37**, 71–84.

Wrighton, S.A. and Stevens, J.C. (1992) The human hepatic cytochromes P450 involved in drug metabolism. *Crit. Rev. Toxicol.* **22**, 1–21.

Ziegler, D.M. (1991) Unique properties of the enzymes of detoxication. *Drug Metab. Disp.* **19**, 847–852.

A list of useful web sites is included at the end of Chapters 2 and 3.

2 ENZYMOLOGY AND MOLECULAR MECHANISMS OF DRUG METABOLISM REACTIONS

LEARNING OBJECTIVES

At the end of this chapter, you should be able to:
• Understand the role of metabolism in the excretion of drugs and xenobiotics
• Describe the structure, function and molecular genetics of the drug-metabolising enzymes
• Appreciate the substrate specificity (with examples) of the drug-metabolising enzymes
• Have a knowledge of the control and interaction of drug metabolism pathways

2.1 INTRODUCTION

As described in Chapter 1, drugs and xenobiotics are transformed by a variety of pathways in two distinct stages. The phase 1 (or functionalisation) reactions serve to introduce a suitable functional group into the drug molecule, thereby changing the drug in most cases to a more polar and hence more readily excretable form. In addition, the product of phase 1 drug metabolism may then act as a substrate for phase 2 metabolism, resulting in conjugation with endogenous compounds, increased water solubility and polarity, and drug elimination/excretion from the body. In a quantitative sense, the liver is the main organ responsible for phase 1 and phase 2 drug metabolism reactions, although this is by no means the only organ involved. Drug localisation, and hence metabolism, in a given tissue is dependent on many factors including the physicochemical properties of the drug (pK_a, lipid solubility and molecular weight), chemical composition of the organ and the presence of specific uptake mechanisms which allow the drug to be concentrated in a particular tissue. As drugs are commonly given several times per day for long periods, it is not surprising that drug binding and metabolism sites become saturated in a given organ. This can then lead to drug diffusion to other sites in the body and may well explain some bizarre side effects observed after prolonged drug treatment. Almost every organ in the body is capable of catalysing drug metabolism reactions, the most prominent of which are the kidney, gastrointestinal tract, gastrointestinal flora, lung, blood, brain, placenta and skin, amongst others.

Most of our fundamental knowledge on the molecular mechanisms of drug metabolism has been derived from studies on the liver. Although the molecular mechanisms of drug metabolism reactions can be studied at many levels of integration, including the intact organism, perfused liver, liver slices and hepatocyte cell cultures, most of our current knowledge has been derived from studies on isolated, subcellular hepatocyte organelles and isolated enzymes and cloned genes.

Table 2.1 Morphological and biochemical characteristics of the hepatic endoplasmic reticulum (ER)

1. Membranes are 50–80 Ångströms in transverse plane.

2. ER occupies approximately 15% of total hepatocyte volume.

3. Volume of ER is 250% of nuclear and 65% of mitochondrial volumes.

4. Surface area of ER is ×37 of plasma membrane and ×9 of outer mitochondrial membrane.

5. ER of one hepatocyte has approximately 13×10^6 attached ribosomes.

6. ER contains 19% total protein, 48% total phospholipid and 58% of total RNA of rat hepatocyte.

7. ER membrane consists of 70% protein, 30% lipid, the majority of which is phospholipid, i.e. approximately 23 molecules of phospholipid per protein molecule.

8. Phospholipid of ER comprises 55% phosphatidylcholine, 20–25% phosphatidylethanolamine, 5–10% phosphatidylserine, 5–10% phosphatidylinositol and 4–7% sphingomyelin.

9. The fatty acid content of above phospholipids mainly consist of palmitic, palmitoleic, stearic, oleic, linoleic and arachidonic acids.

10. ER also contains cholesterol (0.6 mg/g liver), triglycerides (0.5 mg/g liver) and small amounts of cholesterol esters, free fatty acids and vitamin K.

11. ER contains proteins that are 2% carbohydrate by weight containing the neutral sugars mannose and galactose.

12. ER can be induced by many drugs including phenobarbitone resulting in proliferation of protein and phospholipid.

Table 2.2 Enzymatic activities observed in hepatic endoplasmic reticulum

1. Synthesis of triglycerides, phosphatides, glycolipids and plasmalogens.

2. Metabolism of plasmalogens.

3. Fatty acid metabolism including oxidation, elongation and desaturation.

4. Cholesterol and steroid biosynthesis and metabolism.

5. Cytochrome P450-dependent drug oxidations, including hydroxylations, side chain oxidations, deamination, N- and S-oxidation and desulfuration.

6. L-Ascorbic acid synthesis.

7. Aryl- and steroid-sulfatases.

8. Epoxide hydrolase.

9. Cytochrome b_5.

10. NADH-cytochrome b_5 reductase.

11. NADPH-cytochrome c(P450) reductase.

12. Glucose-6-phosphatase.

13. UDP–glucuronosyltransferase.

14. L-Amino acid oxidase.

15. Azo reductase.

16. Cholesterol esterase.

17. 5′-Nucleotidase.

18. Lipid peroxidase.

19. 11β- and 17β-hydroxysteroid dehydrogenases.

With respect to drug metabolism reactions, two subcellular organelles are quantitatively the most important, namely the endoplasmic reticulum (or microsomes) and the cytosol (or soluble cell sap fraction). The phase 1 oxidative enzymes are almost exclusively localised in the endoplasmic reticulum, along with the phase 2 enzyme, glucuronosyl transferase. In contrast, other phase 2 enzymes, including the glutathione-S-transferases and the sulfate-conjugating enzymes are predominantly found in the cytoplasm. In the intact cell, the endoplasmic reticulum consists of a continuous network of filamentous membranes and physical disruption thereof results in the formation of 'microsomes' (literally small bodies). The microsomal fraction of cells is an operational term used to describe the pinched-off and vesiculated fragments of the original endoplasmic reticulum that retain the majority of enzyme activity. As shown in Tables 2.1 and 2.2, the hepatic endoplasmic reticulum serves many important functional roles in addition to drug metabolism reactions. Thus, drug metabolism reactions should not be considered in isolation, but rather as part of a system integrated with other physiological/ biochemical functions.

Based on information gained from studies on intact microsomal membranes, cytosolic fractions and purified enzyme components, it is the purpose of this chapter to clarify, on a cellular and molecular level, the enzyme-catalysed reactions of drug metabolism. This has been the subject of intense scientific research in recent years and the interested reader is referred to the section on further reading for more detailed information.

2.2 CYTOCHROME P450-DEPENDENT MIXED-FUNCTION OXIDATION REACTIONS

The most intensively studied drug metabolism reaction is the cytochrome P450-catalysed mixed-function oxidase (MFO) reaction. This reaction catalyses the oxidation of literally thousands of structurally diverse drugs and chemicals, whose only common feature appears to be a reasonably high degree of lipid solubility (lipophilicity). The MFO reaction is characterised by the following stoichiometry:

$$NADPH\ H^+ + O_2 + RH \xrightarrow{\text{Cytochrome P450}} NADP^+ + H_2O + ROH$$

where RH represents an oxidisable drug substrate and ROH is the hydroxylated metabolite, the overall reaction being catalysed by the enzyme cytochrome P450. During the MFO reaction, reducing equivalents derived from NADPH H^+ are consumed and one atom of molecular oxygen is incorporated into the metabolite, and the other atom of oxygen is reduced to the level of water. Studies using $^{18}O_2$ have unequivocally shown that the source of oxygen in the metabolite is derived from molecular oxygen (and not water). In addition to hydroxylation reactions, cytochrome P450 catalyses the N-, O- and S-dealkylation of many drugs (see Chapter 1). These heteroatom dealkylation reactions can be considered as a specialised form of hydroxylation reaction, in that the initial event is a carbon-based hydroxylation as described in Chapter 1.

2.2.1 Components of the MFO system

Cytochrome P450

Cytochrome P450 is the terminal oxidase component of an electron transfer system present in the endoplasmic reticulum responsible for the oxidation of almost all drugs, and is classified as a haem-containing enzyme (a haemoprotein) with iron protoporphyrin IX as the prosthetic group (Figure 2.1). This prosthetic group is common to other haemoproteins, but with substantially different biological functions, such as haemoglobin and myoglobin (oxygen transport proteins), catalase (splits hydrogen peroxide to oxygen and water) and horseradish peroxidase, cytochrome c peroxidase (uses hydrogen peroxide as an oxidant) and mitochondrial redox cytochromes (plays a role in electron and reducing equivalent transport). As we have seen, cytochrome P450 mainly acts to hydroxylate organic compounds and the reason for this diversity of haemoprotein function, particularly in cytochrome P450, is due, in part, to the nature of the fifth and sixth ligands to the protein. This ligation to the haem iron is extremely important in determining the electron distribution in the haem group, hence its behaviour in chemical (enzymatic) reactions (see the discussion on the cytochrome P450 spin state in Section 2.2.2). Spectrally, cytochrome P450 is a 'b'-type cytochrome, but an unusual one in that it readily reacts with small molecular weight ligands, it exists as an equilibrium mixture of both low and high spin forms and the spectral absorbance maximum of the ferrous–carbon monoxide adduct is 450 nm, as compared to around 420 nm for the majority of other haemoproteins. These unusual properties of cytochrome P450 are largely dictated by the cysteinyl fifth ligand to the haem iron.

Cytochrome P450 is not a single enzyme, but rather consists of a family of closely related isoforms embedded in the membrane of the endoplasmic reticulum, and exists as multiple forms of monomeric molecular weight of approximately 45 000–55 000 daltons. The haem of cytochrome P450 is non-covalently bound to the apoprotein and the name 'cytochrome P450' is derived from the fact that the

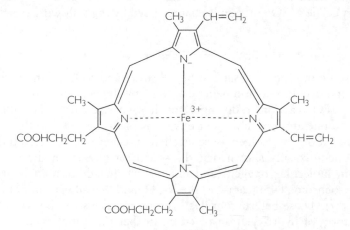

Figure 2.1 Structure of ferric protoporphyrin IX, the prosthetic group of cytochrome P450.

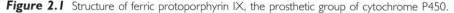

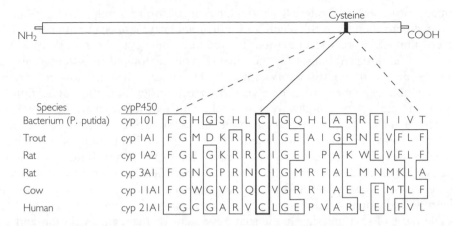

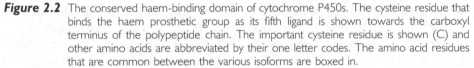

Figure 2.2 The conserved haem-binding domain of cytochrome P450s. The cysteine residue that binds the haem prosthetic group as its fifth ligand is shown towards the carboxyl terminus of the polypeptide chain. The important cysteine residue is shown (C) and other amino acids are abbreviated by their one letter codes. The amino acid residues that are common between the various isoforms are boxed in.

cytochrome (or *pigment*) exhibits a spectral absorbance maximum (Soret peak) at 450 nm when reduced (Fe^{2+}-haem) and complexed with carbon monoxide. The haemoprotein serves as the locus for oxygen binding/activation (and the binding site for some, but not all, drugs) and in conjunction with its associated flavoprotein reductase (NADPH-cytochrome P450 reductase, see below) undergoes cyclic reduction/oxidation of the haem iron that is mandatory for its catalytic activity.

Cumulative historical evidence and more recent studies on the experimental manipulation of cytochrome P450 genes are beginning to yield fascinating information on the structural and functional domains of the P450s. For example, particular regions of the proteins are thought to involve a membrane insertion sequence, a binding site for cytochrome b_5, sites of phosphorylation by cAMP-dependent protein kinases, several substrate-binding sites, an NADPH-cytochrome P450 binding site and a highly conserved region near the carboxyl terminal responsible for haem binding via the invariant cysteine residue. While many of these domains are still to be fully clarified, one fact that is absolutely clear is the presence of the invariant haem-binding segment (via a cysteine residue) of approximately 15 amino acid residues, a sequence that is conserved in all cytochromes P450 studied to date, ranging from bacteria through lower mammals to man (Figure 2.2).

Multiple forms of cytochrome P450 and nomenclature
Ever since its initial purification and isolation in a catalytically competent form in the late 1960s, many studies have emphasised that cytochrome P450 exists as multiple forms derived from separate and distinct genes. To date, over 800 different cytochrome P450 genes have been isolated and completely sequenced, this number encompassing all of the major phyla including the animalia, plantae,

fungi, protoctista and monera (bacteria) kingdoms. Unfortunately, this has resulted in much confusion as to the identity of individual enzymes because no commonly agreed nomenclature system existed. In fact, individual cytochromes P450 would have several different names for the same enzyme if isolated in different laboratories – clearly an unsatisfactory situation. However, with the advent of gene cloning, the refinement of gene sequencing technology and the application of molecular biology techniques to cytochrome P450 structure analysis, the 1980s witnessed an explosion in the isolation and sequencing of cDNAs encoding multiple forms of the haemoprotein. This rapid accumulation of full-length cytochrome P450 amino acid sequences (predicted from open reading frames of the cognate cDNA nucleotide sequences) then allowed the development of a coherent nomenclature system which has now been universally accepted and uniquely identifies individual P450s.

The basis of this unifying nomenclature system is divergent evolution and sequence similarity between the cytochromes P450, resulting in the sub-classification of P450s into gene families and gene sub-families. Specifically, a cytochrome P450 sequence from one gene family is defined as having less than 40% sequence similarity to that from any other family. Put another way, within a given cytochrome P450 gene family, all the component genes in that family are greater than 40% identical in their sequence to each other. Individual gene families are further sub-divided into gene sub-families where the nomenclature dictates that two cytochromes P450 belong to the same gene sub-family when they are 70% (or greater) similar in their sequence. Hence CYP3A4 (CYP for cytochrome P450) uniquely describes only one particular gene encoding a specific protein, and is the fourth gene to have been completely sequenced in the 3A sub-family. The next gene to have been sequenced in the CYP3A sub-family is termed CYP3A5 and so forth. The total number of cytochromes P450 is monitored and updated on several web sites and has increased from 65 in 1987, through 221 in 1993 to approximately 800 in 2001. It should be

Table 2.3 Functions of the cytochrome P450 families

P450 family	Function
CYP1–CYP3	Drug, xenobiotic and steroid metabolism
CYP4	Fatty acid, prostaglandin, leukotriene metabolism
CYP5	Thromboxane synthesis
CYP7	Cholesterol 7α-hydroxylation
CYP11	Cholesterol side chain cleavage + steroid 11β hydroxylase
CYP17	Steroid 17α-hydroxylation
CYP19	Aromatisation of steroids
CYP21	Steroid 21-hydroxylase
CYP24	Vitamin D hydroxylation
CYP27	Cholesterol 27-hydroxylase

Adapted from Smith, D. et al. (1998) Xenobiotica **28**, 1129–1165

noted that this nomenclature is based on sequence information and does not encompass any classification/description of substrate specificities or catalytic activities, although some broad generalisations can be made (Table 2.3). For a more detailed discussion of this nomenclature, the interested reader is referred to the lists of further reading and web sites at the end of this chapter.

Human liver cytochromes P450

The above genetic approach to the structure, function and regulation of cytochrome P450s has enabled considerable progress in their characterisation from human gene libraries, thus obviating the need for scarce human tissue as a source for purifying and characterising individual enzymes. Over 50 human cytochromes P450 have now been isolated, unequivocally identified and characterised to date, including the steroid hydroxylases (e.g. CYP11A1 and CYP21A2) and the major human liver drug-metabolising cytochromes P450 including CYP1A2, CYP2A6, CYP2E1, CYP2C8/9/18/19, CYP2D6 and CYP3A4/5/7 (Figure 2.3).

The CYP3As are quantitatively the major sub-family expressed in the majority of human livers (approximately 30% of the total) and consist of three forms, namely CYP3A4, CYP3A5 and CYP3A7. CYP3A7 is the major foetal form and is essentially switched off after birth, whereupon CYP3A4 is the major form expressed thereafter (in all age groups). CYP3A5 is polymorphically expressed in approximately 50% of human livers; its substrate specificity parallels that of CYP3A4 but it is generally less active in drug oxidation than CYP3A4. It should be emphasised that the major human liver form, CYP3A4, exhibits a considerable inter-individual variation in expression in the human population by one to two orders of magnitude.

The specific reasons for inter-individual variation in CYP3A4 levels are presently unclear, but hepatic levels of CYP3A4 expression are highly dependent on prior chemical exposure (drug therapy, dietary components and environmental chemicals), which can produce increased or decreased levels of expression/activity (termed induction and inhibition, respectively, as described in detail in Chapter 3), thus potentially contributing to the inter-individual variability. Another aspect of inter-individual variability in CYP3A4 levels is the possibility of genetic variation between individuals, a topic that has been the subject of much investigation but it is only very recently that the molecular genetics of this phenomenon are beginning to unfold. For example, sequencing of the 13 exons and the 5'-flanking region (promoter) of the CYP3A4 gene in Finnish, Chinese (Taiwan) and black populations has been investigated. It turns out that 2.7% of the Finnish population studied have a heterozygotic allelic variant of CYP3A4 (termed CYP3A4*2) which has a single base change in exon 7 of the coding gene, the mutation not being detected in either the black or the Chinese populations. This results in a change of the serine amino acid residue 222 in CYP3A4 to a proline residue. As proline is a known helix-breaker in proteins, it would be anticipated that this change may cause a perturbation of CYP3A4 structure and hence its ability to metabolise its cognate substrates. To address this possibility, full length wild type and mutant CYP3A4 enzymes were generated from their corresponding cDNAs and the enzyme activities towards nifedipine oxidation examined. As shown in Table 2.4,

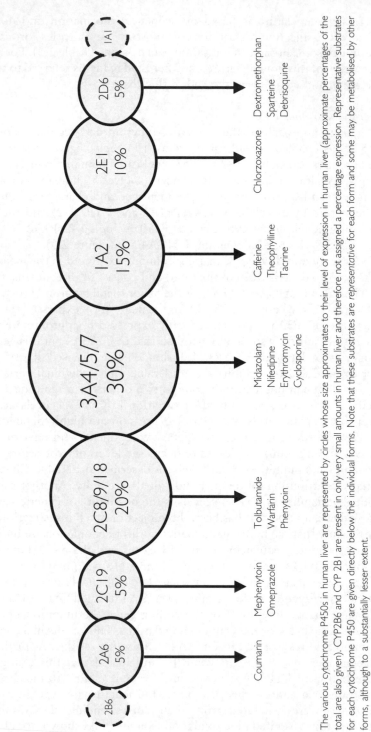

Figure 2.3 Human liver cytochrome P450s and their representative substrates.

The various cytochrome P450s in human liver are represented by circles whose size approximates to their level of expression in human liver (approximate percentages of the total are also given). CYP2B6 and CYP 2B1 are present in only very small amounts in human liver and therefore not assigned a percentage expression. Representative substrates for each cytochrome P450 are given directly below the individual forms. Note that these substrates are representative for each form and some may be metabolised by other forms, although to a substantially lesser extent.

Table 2.4 A mutation in the CYP3A4 gene alters nifedipine oxidation

	Enzyme	
	Wild type (CYP3A4)	**Mutant (CYP3A4*2)**
V_{max} (min^{-1})	36	23
K_m (μM)	2	11
Intrinsic clearance	18	2
(V_{max}/K_m) (min$^{-1} \cdot \mu$M)		

Adapted from Sata, F. et al. (2000) *Pharmacogenetics and Genomics* **67**, 48–56.

in comparison to the active CYP3A4 wild type, the CYP3A4 mutant exhibited a decreased capacity to metabolise nifedipine (a drug used in the treatment of hypertension and prophylaxis of angina) and therefore provides, in part, a genetic basis for inter-individual variation in CYP3A4 expression and hence the ability to metabolise drugs.

Preliminary evidence is emerging for other functional mutations in the CYP3A4 gene in a Chinese population with three additional point mutations/insertions. These have been termed CYP3A4*4 [Ile118Val], CYP3A4*5 [Pro218Arg] and CYP3A4*6, where an A_{17776} insertion produces a frame shift resulting in a premature stop codon in exon 9. These mutations were matched against the urinary ratio of 6β-hydroxycortisol : free cortisol ratio (a measure of *in vivo* CYP3A4 activity) and, in all cases, the mutations reduced the ratio by approximately half, not inconsistent with the conclusion that these mutations produce functional consequences in the CYP3A4 gene.

Similarly, another major human liver cytochrome P450, CYP2D6, exhibits considerable polymorphism in the human population and is responsible for the poor or extensive metaboliser phenotype towards debrisoquine (a cardiac drug) and many other clinical drugs in use today (see Chapter 7 for a fuller description of this phenomenon).

The recent publication of the draft sequence of the complete human genome has revealed that mutations (single-nucleotide polymorphisms or SNPs) occur approximately every 300–1000 nucleotides. Considering that the human genome consists of approximately three billion nucleotides, containing nearly 150 000 coding genes, the possibility of SNPs occurring in a functionally crucial part of a drug-metabolising enzyme are theoretically relatively high. Thus the next few years are almost certainly guaranteed to see an explosion in our knowledge of human pharmacogenetics, thereby providing a coherent explanation of why individuals respond differently to drugs, in both a pharmacological and a toxicological sense. In a broader sense, the Human Genome Mapping Project and the functional genomics arising therefrom will mean that the fourth edition of this text will have a radically different complexion.

The ever-increasing number of cytochrome P450 sequences has also stimulated computer-based molecular modelling of their tertiary structures. This modelling has been facilitated by the crystallisation and high resolution X-ray crystal structure of the soluble bacterial cytochromes P450 from CYP101 (*Pseudomonas putida*) and CYP 102 (*Bacillus megaterium*). Thus, by using the crystal structures of these bacterial cytochromes P450 as a template, other cytochromes P450 can be modelled, based on comparative sequence similarities. Because almost all of the mammalian cytochromes P450 are membrane-bound (and therefore inherently very difficult to crystallise), little information is available on the three-dimensional structure of eukaryotic cytochromes P450. However, recent work on the crystallisation of a fragment of the mammalian, membrane-bound CYP2C5 enzyme represents a substantial step forward in molecular modelling and hence our understanding of the structure and function of eukaryotic cytochrome P450s.

NADPH-cytochrome P450 reductase

NADPH-cytochrome P450 reductase is a flavin-containing enzyme, a flavoprotein consisting of one mole of flavin mononucleotide (FMN) and one mole of flavin adenine nucleotide (FAD) per mole of protein (see Figure 2.4 for structures of these flavins). This makes NADPH-cytochrome P450 reductase unusual as most

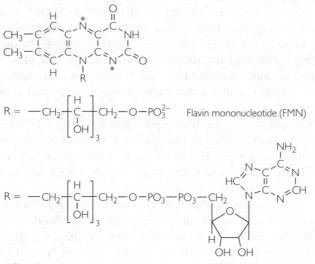

Flavin mononucleotide (FMN)

Flavin adenine dinucleotide (FAD)

* Site of reduction

Figure 2.4 Structures of FAD and FMN, the prosthetic groups of NADPH-cytochrome P450 reductase.

other flavoproteins have only FAD or FMN as their prosthetic group. The flavoprotein is sometimes referred to as NADPH-cytochrome c reductase because of the well-established ability of the enzyme to artificially reduce cytochrome c (an artificial electron acceptor in this instance) in the presence of NADPH H^+. However, because cytochrome c is a mitochondrial haemoprotein and not expressed in the endoplasmic reticulum, the correct terminology for this enzyme is NADPH-cytochrome P450 reductase, in that cytochrome P450 is the endogenous acceptor of reducing equivalents from the reductase. The enzyme has a monomeric molecular weight of approximately 78 000 daltons and exists in close association with cytochrome P450 in the endoplasmic reticulum membrane. In addition to cytochrome P450, NADPH-cytochrome P450 reductase is an essential component of the MFO system responsible for drug oxidation in that the flavoprotein transfers reducing equivalents (essential for the catalytic activity of cytochrome P450, see below) from NADPH H^+ to cytochrome P450 as

NADPH H^+ ⟶ FAD (NADPH-cytochrome P450 reductase) FMN ⟶ cytochrome P450

The need for an intermediary electron transfer protein is readily appreciated in light of the fact that NADPH H^+ is a two-electron donor and cytochrome P450 is a (2×1)-electron acceptor. Accordingly, NADPH-cytochrome P450 reductase is thought to act as a 'transducer' of reducing equivalents by accepting electrons from NADPH H^+ and transferring them sequentially (one at a time) to cytochrome P450. The precise redox biochemistry (oxidation/reduction) of NADPH-cytochrome P450 reductase during cytochrome P450-dependent drug oxidation is not fully understood, as the redox biochemistry of the two flavins is complex (Figure 2.5 and Table 2.5), although there is very strong evidence to support the role of FAD as the acceptor of reducing equivalents from NADPH H^+ and FMN as the donating flavin to cytochrome P450 during drug metabolism.

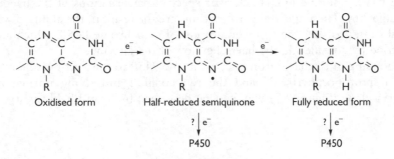

Oxidised form · Half-reduced semiquinone · Fully reduced form

Figure 2.5 Flavin reduction.

Table 2.5 Redox biochemistry of the two flavin prosthetic groups present in NADPH-cytochrome P450 reductase

$F_1 + H^· \rightleftharpoons F_1H^·$, $E_m = -110\,mV$	$E_m = -190\,mV$
$F_1H^· = H^· \rightleftharpoons F_1H_2$, $E_m = -270\,mV$	
$F_2 + H^· \rightleftharpoons F_2H^·$, $E_m = -290\,mV$	$E_m = -320\,mV$
$F_2H^· = H^· \rightleftharpoons F_2H_2$, $E_m = -365\,mV$	

Abbreviations used: F_1, high potential flavin (probably FMN); F_2, low potential flavin (probably FAD); E_m, mid-point redox potential.

Role of lipids in drug oxidation

Early studies on the resolution and reconstitution of MFO activity in drug oxidation have shown the requirement of a heat-stable, lipid component. This component was originally identified as phosphatidylcholine and later studies demonstrated that the fatty acid composition of the phospolipid is critical in determining the functional reconstitution of MFO activity. The precise mode of action of lipids in the MFO reaction is still a subject for conjecture, but it has been suggested that lipid may either facilitate substrate binding, electron transfer or provide a 'template' for the essential interaction of cytochrome P450 and NADPH-cytochrome P450 reductase molecules.

2.2.2 Catalytic cycle of cytochrome P450

As mentioned above, cytochrome P450 is both the substrate- and oxygen-binding locus of the MFO reaction. The central features of the cytochrome P450 catalytic cycle are the ability of the haem iron to undergo cyclic oxidation/reduction in conjunction with substrate binding and oxygen activation, as outlined in Figure 2.6.

Step 1. This is a relatively well characterised step and involves drug binding to the oxidised (ferric, Fe^{3+}) form of cytochrome P450. Early experiments in the late 1960s categorised drug binding into three types, namely Type I, Type II and Reverse Type I. At the time, these classifications were arbitrarily made on the basis of the observed drug-induced changes in the absorbance spectrum of cytochrome P450, resulting in characteristic spectral perturbations of the haemoprotein (Table 2.6). These spectral perturbations are the result of the ability of various drug substrates to shift the spin equilibrium of cytochrome P450, which are best understood by considering the haem ligation of the enzyme.

The bonding of the haem iron of cytochrome P450 to the four pyrrole nitrogen atoms of protoporphyrin IX and the two axial ligands lying normal to the porphyrin plane (Figure 2.7) may best be described by ligand field theory. Thus,

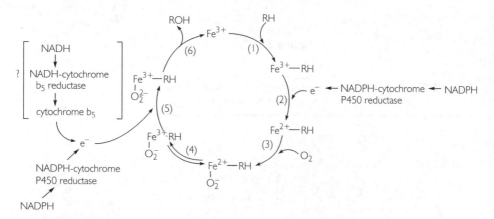

Figure 2.6 Catalytic cycle of cytochrome P450. RH represents the drug substrate and ROH the corresponding hydroxylated metabolite.

Table 2.6 Spectral interaction of drugs and other xenobiotics with cytochrome P450[a]

Type I	Type II	Reverse Type I
Aldrin	Aniline	Acetanilide
Aminopyrine	Amphetamine	Butanol
Benzphetamine	Cyanide	Diallyl barbituric acid
Caffeine	Dapsone	Ethanol
Chlorpromazine	Desdimethylimipramine	Methanol
Cocaine	Imidazole	Phenacetin
DDT	Metyrapone	Rotenone
Diphenylhydantoin	Nicotinamide	Theophylline
Ethylmorphine	Nicotine	Warfarin
Halothane	p-Phenetidine	
Hexobarbital	Pyridine	
Imipramine		
Phenobarbitone		
Propranolol		
Testosterone		

[a] Spectral changes of cytochrome P450 induced by xenobiotics have the following UV/visible characteristics in difference spectrum:
  Type I, absorption peak at 385–390 nm and trough at approximately 420 nm.
  Type II, absorption peak at 425–435 nm and trough at 390–405 nm.
  Reverse type I (sometimes termed Modified Type II), absorption peak at 420 nm and trough at 388–390 nm.
  Derifved from Schenkman, J. et al. (1981) Pharmacol. Ther. **12**, 43.

upon coordination of the ferric haem iron with these six ligands in an octahedral complex, the electrons occupying the d-orbitals of the ferric iron (which are energetically degenerate in the free ion) are, as a result of differences in their spatial arrangement, subjected to differential electron repulsion by the lone pair electrons of the ligands. Thus the electrons occupying the d_{z^2} and $d_{x^2-y^2}$ orbitals (the lobes of which collectively exhibit octahedral symmetry and are oriented

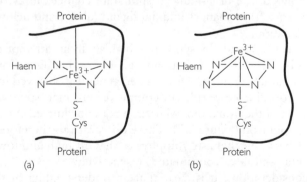

Figure 2.7 Haem iron coordination in cytochrome P450. (a) Hexa-coordinated, low spin P450 with in-plane iron. (b) Penta-coordinated, high-spin P450 with out-of-plane iron. Note that the fifth ligand is a cysteine residue from the apoprotein and that cytochrome P450 exists as an equilibrium mixture of low-spin (6-coordinated) and high-spin (5-coordinated) forms, this equilibrium being perturbed by the presence of a drug. See text for detailed discussion of ligation and spin states.

along the ligand bond axis) experience a greater electron repulsion than electrons occupying the d_{xy}, d_{yz} and d_{xz} orbitals (lying between the bond axes). This results in a splitting of the energy levels of the ferric d-orbitals as shown in Figure 2.8. The magnitude of the energy separation between the two higher energy orbitals (e_g) and the three lower energy orbitals (t_{2g}) is called the crystal field splitting (or stabilisation) energy, termed ΔE, and is a function of the strength of the ligand to ferric d-orbital repulsion forces and thus the ligand field strength. The magnitude of ΔE has profound effects upon the distribution of the ferric d electrons. Thus, if ΔE is greater than the energetic instability (C) resulting from electron–electron repulsion in a spin-paired d-orbital, then a low spin d-electron configuration of $S = 1/2$ (one unpaired d-electron) results. Conversely, if C is greater than ΔE a maximum paramagnetic configuration of $S = 5/2$ (five unpaired d-electrons) results (Figure 2.8).

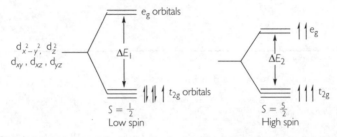

Figure 2.8 d-Orbital electron distribution in the low- and high-spin states of cytochrome P450.

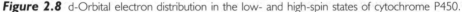

From this simplistic description, it is readily seen that a change in the spin state of the ferric haem iron is associated with a change in ΔE which is envisaged as arising due to quantitative or qualitative alterations in the ligands coordinated to the haem iron. Since it is absolutely required that the four equatorial iron to pyrrole nitrogen bonds remain bonded, the drug-induced spin state changes in cytochrome P450 almost certainly arise from changes in axial ligand (above and below the plane of the haem) coordination.

Much effort has been made by synthetic chemists in an attempt to understand the relationship between the spin state and geometric configuration of synthetic metal–porphyrin model complexes. It has been generally observed in these studies that most penta-coordinated porphyrin complexes are high spin with an out-of-plane displacement of the iron atom, whereas hexa-coordinated complexes exhibit an in-plane, low spin iron (Figure 2.7). These observations therefore lend support to the dogma of haem biochemistry/biophysics that all high and low spin haemoproteins are penta- and hexa-coordinated, respectively.

From such considerations, it is clear that an understanding of the immediate haem environment of cytochrome P450, and in particular the nature of the axial ligands, is crucial in understanding its mechanism of catalysis. The importance of axial ligands as determinants of haemoprotein function is further substantiated when one considers that cytochrome P450 (an MFO enzyme), haemoglobin (an oxygen carrier), peroxidases and catalase all contain protoporphyrin IX as their common prosthetic group, yet all of them perform substantially different biological functions.

Most cytochromes P450 exist in the predominantly low spin state with a ferric Soret absorbance at around 418 nm. When certain drug substrates bind to the low spin form, they usually bind to the protein part of the molecule and change the conformation and hence the ligation of the haem prosthetic group with the protein. These drugs are termed Type I substrates and include hexobarbital and benzphetamine. This results in a shift of the spin equilibrium of cytochrome P450 towards the high spin form, resulting in a characteristic spectral change (termed Type I), with an absorbance maximum at around 390 nm and a minimum at around 420 nm in the difference spectrum (Figure 2.9). This difference spectrum arises due to the increase in absorbance at 390 nm (high spin form) and a decrease in absorbance at 420 nm (low spin form) on the binding of a Type I substrate. Thus, Type I substrates can be considered as those that modulate the spin equilibrium of cytochrome P450.

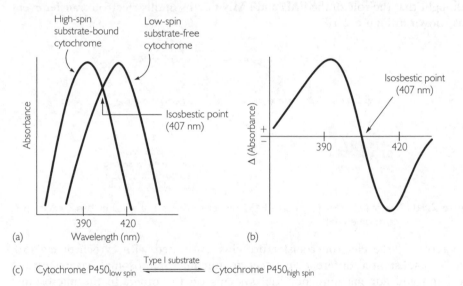

Figure 2.9 Spectral interaction of a type I substrate with cytochrome P450. (a) Influence of substrate on the absolute absorbance spectrum of cytochrome P450. Note the increase in absorbance at 390 nm and decrease at 420 nm upon substrate addition. (b) Substrate-induced type I difference spectrum. Note that the spectral changes result from the absorbance changes in (a). (c) Influence of a type I substrate on the spin equilibrium of cytochrome P450. Note that type I substrates shift the spin equilibrium to the high spin form.

In contrast to Type I substrates, Type II substrates are mainly nitrogenous bases and are thought to ligate directly to the haem iron of cytochrome P450 (via the lone pair electrons on the nitrogen atom), resulting in a hexa-coordinated, low spin haemoprotein.

An important *functional* consequence of these drug-induced spin state changes in cytochrome P450 is that the spin state shift is associated with changes in the midpoint redox potential (ability to be reduced) of the haemoprotein. For example, a shift in the spin state of both bacterial and mammalian cytochromes P450 towards the high spin form is associated with a shift in the midpoint redox potential to a more positive value (and hence more readily reducible). This spin–redox coupling phenomenon is very likely to be of functional significance when one considers that the first one-electron reduction of ferric cytochrome P450 (step 2) by NADPH-cytochrome P450 reductase represents the committed step in cytochrome P450-dependent catalysis. A substrate-induced shift in the haemoprotein midpoint redox potential to a more positive value results in a greater electromotive force for subsequent facile electron transfer (reduction) between the flavoprotein and the cytochrome.

Step 2. This involves the first electron reduction of substrate-bound ferric (Fe^{3+}) cytochrome P450 to the ferrous (Fe^{2+}) form of the haemoprotein. The reducing equivalent necessary for this reduction is initially derived from NADPH H^+ and is transferred by the flavoprotein, NADPH-cytochrome P450 reductase. It is thought that the role of the FAD and FMN flavins in this electron transfer event is as shown in Figure 2.10.

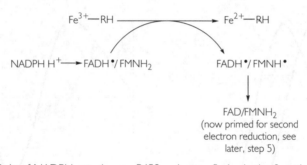

Figure 2.10 Role of NADPH-cytochrome P450 reductase flavins in the first electron reduction of cytochrome P450.

In terms of the electron transfer proteins associated with cytochrome P450, there is a substantial difference between mammalian microsomal systems on the one hand and adrenal mitochondrial systems on the other. In the microsomal system electron transfer occurs in the sequence

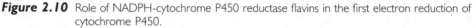

as described above, whereas there is an additional requirement for an iron-sulfur protein in the mitochondrial system, namely adrenodoxin as

NADPH H^+ ⟶ NADPH-adrenodoxin reductase ⟶ adrenodoxin ⟶ cytochrome P450

It should be noted that, unlike microsomal NADPH-cytochrome P450 reductase, adrenal NADPH-adrenodoxin reductase contains only FAD as the flavin prosthetic group. In addition, the adrenal mitochondrial cytochrome P450 is different from its microsomal counterpart in that the former haemoprotein does not readily catalyse the oxidation of drugs. The endogenous roles for the cytochromes P450 have been described in Chapter 1 and a more extensive consideration of the structure and regulation of the cytochromes P450 is presented in Chapter 3.

As mentioned above, the high spin/low spin equilibrium of cytochrome P450 is crucial for this first electron reduction step. However, a fuller understanding of the spin–redox coupling in steps 1 and 2 of the catalytic cycle is not yet complete because of the inherent complexities associated with the redox biochemistry of the electron donor flavoprotein, which contains both FAD and FMN prosthetic groups, and is therefore a potential four-electron carrier (Table 2.5).

Although existing experimental evidence is strongly supportive of spin–redox coupling (with respect to haemoprotein reduction), extrapolations from thermodynamic data (spin state *equilibrium*) to the kinetic situation (one-electron reduction *rate*) have to be treated with some caution. This is primarily because the electromotive force for a redox reaction is a function of both the forward and reverse rate constants for the electron transfer event.

Step 3. This step involves binding of molecular oxygen to the binary ferrous cytochrome P450-substrate complex. This reaction is not well characterised in the mammalian system due to the unstable nature of the oxy-ferrous-substrate complex, but has been spectrally identified in the soluble bacterial system of *Pseudomonas putida* (CYP101, formerly known as $P450_{cam}$ in the old nomenclature, so called because the bacterium grows on camphor as the sole source of carbon and catalyses the 5-exo-hydroxylation of camphor).

Steps 4, 5 and 6. These steps involve putative electron rearrangement, introduction of the second electron and subsequent oxygen insertion into the drug substrate and hydroxylated metabolite release. The precise oxidation states of iron and oxygen in these intermediates are not precisely known. Step 5 involves the input of the second electron, usually derived from NADPH-cytochrome P450 reductase, or alternatively, derived from cytochrome b_5 and its associated flavoprotein reductase (Figure 2.11). Although NADPH-cytochrome P450 is the source of the second-electron donation for the majority of drug oxidation reactions, the cytochrome b_5 system can also perform this function, depending on the particular drug substrate and particular form of cytochrome P450 under consideration. Similarly, step 6 is not well understood and primarily concerns the actual chemical mechanism of oxygen insertion into the substrate, resulting in product (metabolite) formation. However, the prevailing view of the chemistry of metabolite formation involves two steps, namely abstraction of a hydrogen from the substrate (RH) and oxygen rebound as

$$(FeO)^{3+} + RH \longrightarrow (FeOH)^{3+} + R^{\bullet} \longrightarrow Fe^{3+} + ROH$$

A detailed discussion of the inorganic and organic chemistry involved in the latter reaction is outside the scope of this chapter and the interested reader is referred to the further reading section for more detailed information on this topic.

It should be pointed out that, under certain conditions in the presence of particular drug substrates, the catalytic cycle of cytochrome P450 becomes 'uncoupled'. This uncoupling involves dissociation of the utilisation of reducing equivalents

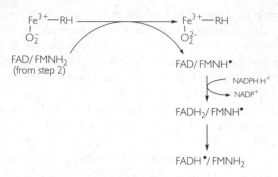

Figure 2.11 Role of NADPH-cytochrome reductase flavins in the second electron reduction of cytochrome P450.

from metabolite formation, resulting in the production of reduced oxygen species (hydrogen peroxide, H_2O_2) instead of stoichiometric metabolite formation as dictated by the MFO reaction described earlier. Accordingly, in producing hydrogen peroxide in an uncoupled system, cytochrome P450 functions as an NADPH-oxidase as

$$O_2 + NADPH\ H^+ \xrightarrow{\text{P450}} H_2O_2 + NADP^+$$

Although the precise source of hydrogen peroxide is not known, it is most likely that it arises from dismutation of the oxygenated cytochrome P450 intermediates produced during the catalytic cycle.

In addition to functioning as an MFO and an NADPH-oxidase, the cytochrome P450's versatility is not exhausted yet and can additionally function as an epoxidase (catalysing the addition of an oxygen across a carbon–carbon double bond) and as a peroxidase (catalysing the cleavage of organic peroxides).

2.3 MICROSOMAL FLAVIN-CONTAINING MONOOXYGENASE

This enzyme was originally called the microsomal mixed-function amine oxidase in view of the fact that many tertiary amines were N-oxidised by this enzyme in a mixed-function oxidase reaction. In the older scientific literature, it was also known as 'Ziegler's enzyme', so called after the scientist who discovered it. However, more recent work has shown that the enzyme additionally catalyses the S-oxidation of organic compounds (Figure 2.12). Accordingly, the enzyme is more appropriately termed the microsomal FAD-containing monooxygenase (usually abbreviated to FMO) and catalyses the following reaction, where RN is an oxidisable, amine-containing substrate and RN–O is the N-oxidised metabolite:

$$NAD(P)H\ H^+ + O_2 + RN \xrightarrow{\text{FMO}} NAD(P)^+ + H_2O + RN–O$$

The FMOs are polymeric proteins exhibiting a monomeric molecular weight of approximately 65 000 daltons and contain one mole of FAD per mole of protein

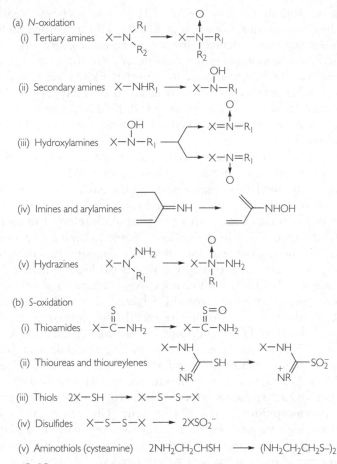

Figure 2.12 Metabolism of xenobiotics by the flavin-containing monooxygenase.

monomer. The enzyme is found in many tissues, with the highest expression being found in the microsomal fraction of the liver. FMO uses either NADH or NADPH as a source of reducing equivalents in the above reaction, although the K_m for NADH is approximately ten times higher than that for NADPH (i.e. NADPH half-saturates the enzyme at one-tenth the concentration of NADH and NADPH is therefore the preferred cofactor). As mentioned above, the FMO catalyses the oxygenation of many nucleophilic organic nitrogen and sulfur compounds, including many drugs such as the phenothiazines, ephedrine, N-methylamphetamine and norcocaine and the thioether- and carbamate-containing pesticides such as Phorate and Thiofanox. This broad substrate specificity, coupled with the wide tissue distribution, additionally suggests the existence of multiple forms (isoforms) of FMO and this is indeed the case.

Like the cytochromes P450, the FMOs are a multi-gene family encoding different enzymes, classified into the five families (FMO1–5), each of which has differing substrate specificities. Specific amino acid regions are conserved in FMOs across species, particularly residues 4–32 and 186–213 which represent the FAD- and NADPH-binding domains, respectively. FMO3 is the major human liver form, which has a broad substrate specificity for drugs and other xenobiotics and whose major role is in detoxification but is also capable of activating some xenobiotics to toxic biological reactive intermediates. In contrast, FMO1 predominates in the liver of most all other species studied to date but is only expressed in low levels in the human liver. Unlike the cytochromes P450, the FMOs are generally refractory to induction by exogenous xenobiotics, but are subject to hormonal and developmental regulation.

Interestingly, it is becoming increasingly recognised that dietary components influence the hepatic and extra-hepatic levels of various FMOs, including indole-3-carbinol (found in cruciferous vegetables), which has recently been shown to dramatically switch off the expression of FMO1 in rat liver and intestine. Related to this dietary aspect is the inborn error of metabolism referred to as Trimethyl-aminuria, or 'Fish Odour Syndrome (FOS)'. Trimethylamine is a normal constituent of the diet and is a pungent and odorous compound (smelling of decayed and rotten fish), but fortunately trimethylamine is oxidised in man by FMO3 to the non-odorous metabolite, trimethylamine N-oxide which is excreted in the urine. However, patients suffering from FOS have FMO-null alleles (termed Ile-66 and Leu-153) which confer a complete inability to detoxify trimethylamine, resulting in the observed FOS syndrome, a particularly distressing condition characterised by a high suicide rate and other psychological aberrations.

Other human genetic polymorphisms in FMO3 have also been identified, including Lys-158, Met-257 and, in *in vitro* experiments, are characterised by a 5- to 100-fold decrease in FMO activity, depending on the particular substrate. Furthermore, other genetic polymorphisms in the FMO3 gene (Glu158Lys and Val257Met) occur at relatively high frequencies in the Caucasian populations studied to date, and may thus result in a compromised ability to metabolise FMO3 substrates.

Based on kinetic and spectral studies, the mechanism of flavin-dependent mono-oxygenation occurs as shown in Figure 2.13. This involves initial flavin reduction (step 1), oxygen binding (step 2), internal electron transfer to oxygen forming the peroxy-flavin complex (step 3), substrate binding (step 4), oxygenated product (metabolite) release (step 5) and dissociation of $NADP^+$ to reform the original oxidised enzyme (step 6). In the absence of an oxidisable substrate, the peroxy-flavin intermediate slowly decomposes, yielding H_2O_2 (step 7). The ordered reaction sequence is summarised in Figure 2.13(b). The peroxy-flavin is a strong electrophile and should therefore be capable of oxidising any nucleophilic compounds, such as N- and S-containing xenobiotics. As already summarised in Figure 2.13, this is indeed the case. However, nucleophilic compounds containing an anionic group are effectively excluded from the active site of the enzyme and it has been suggested that this structural feature serves to exclude the futile oxidation of normal cellular components, since most endogenous nucleophiles contain one or more negatively charged groups.

It should be emphasised that FMO is the only known mammalian flavoprotein hydroxylase, although many bacterial examples are known. In addition, the

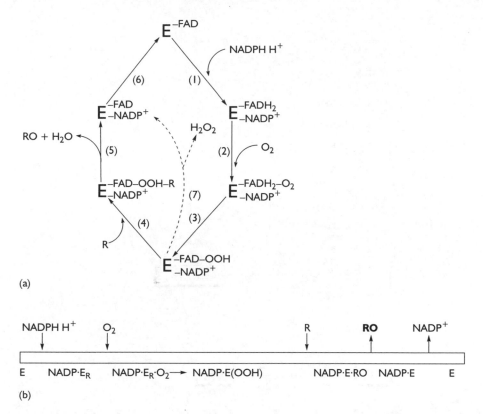

Figure 2.13 Oxidation of N- and S-containing xenobiotics by the microsomal flavin-containing monooxygenase (FMO). Abbreviations used: E-FAD, oxidised enzyme; E-FADH$_2$, reduced enzyme; R, oxidisable substrate; E, oxidised enzyme; E$_R$, reduced enzyme.

reaction mechanism described in Figure 2.13 dictates that substrate binding occurs *after* pyridine nucleotide reduction, again an unusual feature of this enzyme (cf. cytochrome P450).

2.4 PROSTAGLANDIN SYNTHETASE-DEPENDENT CO-OXIDATION OF DRUGS

Prostaglandin synthetase is an enzyme present in almost all mammalian types and catalyses the oxidation of arachidonic acid to prostaglandin H$_2$, the precursor to other physiologically important prostaglandins, thromboxanes and prostacyclin. The enzyme has two distinct catalytic functions, namely fatty acid cyclooxygenase activity, forming prostaglandin G$_2$ as an intermediate, and hydroperoxidase activity, reducing prostaglandin G$_2$ to prostaglandin H$_2$. As shown in Figure 2.14(a), drugs and other xenobiotics are co-oxidised during arachidonic acid metabolism by prostaglandin synthetase, a biotransformation related to the hydroperoxidase component of the enzyme. Several drugs are capable of undergoing this co-oxidation reaction, including aminopyrine, benzphetamine, oxyphenbutazone and

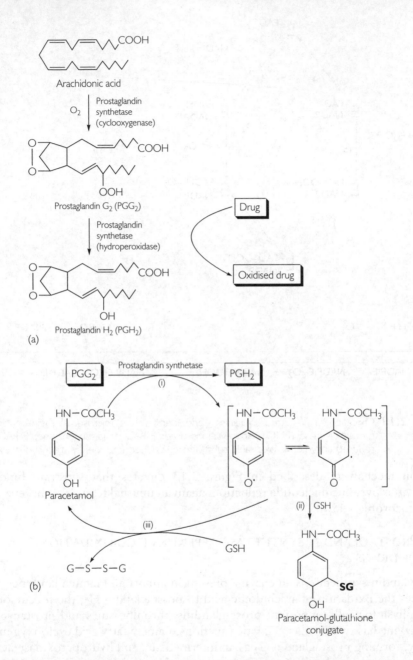

Figure 2.14 Co-oxidation of drugs by prostaglandin synthetase. (a) Role of prostaglandin synthetase in drug oxidations. (b) Postulated mechanism of the prostaglandin synthetase-mediated metabolism of paracetamol. Abbreviations used: GSH, glutathione; G-S-S-G, oxidised glutathione.

paracetamol as well as chemical carcinogens such as benzidine, benzo(*a*)pyrene, benzo(*a*)pyrene-7,8-dihydrodiol, 7,12-dimethylbenzanthracene and *N*-[4-(5-nitro-2-furyl) 2-thiazolyl] formamide.

Furthermore, drugs such as paracetamol appear to undergo a radical-mediated reaction resulting in the formation of glutathione conjugation of the drug (Figure 2.14(b)). This reaction probably involves a one-electron oxidation resulting in hydrogen abstraction to yield the phenoxy radical of paracetamol (step i). This radical then has one of two fates. Firstly, the phenoxy radical tautomerises, forming the carbon-centred quinone radical which can then react with cellular glutathione (the tripeptide Glu–Cys–Gly), forming the glutathione conjugate (step ii). Alternatively, the phenoxy radical may by reduced by glutathione, reforming the parent paracetamol (step iii). Support is given to this reaction mechanism by the rapid depletion of glutathione during the reaction. It should be pointed out that paracetamol also undergoes substantial metabolism by the cytochrome P450 system as described earlier, although the relative contributions made by these two enzyme systems to the overall *in vivo* metabolism of paracetamol is at present unknown. Certainly, the prostaglandin synthetase co-oxidation of certain drugs is a significant metabolic pathway and could conceivably play a substantial role in those tissues that are comparatively rich in prostaglandin synthetase and relatively low in MFO activity, such as the kidney, urinary bladder, renal medulla, skin and lung.

2.5 REDUCTIVE DRUG METABOLISM

As with the oxidative drug metabolism reactions described above, the microsomal mixed-function oxidase system makes a significant contribution to reductive drug metabolism pathways and, as shown in Table 2.7, many different chemical groups are susceptible to enzymatic reduction. Although our collective knowledge of

Table 2.7 Examples of reductive drug metabolism

Reduced chemical group	Reaction	Example
Nitro	$-NO_2 \longrightarrow -NH-OH$	Nitrofurantoin Chloramphenicol
Nitroso	$-N=O \longrightarrow -NH-OH$	Nitroso amantadine
Tertiary amine oxides	$-N \rightarrow O \longrightarrow N-OH$	N-oxides of imipramine, tiaramide and indicine
Hydroxylamine	$-NH-OH \longrightarrow -NH_2$	N-hydroxyphentermine
Azo	$R^1-N=N-R^2 \longrightarrow R^1-NH_2 + R^2-NH_2$	Prontosil, Amaranth
Quinone	quinone $\longrightarrow$ semiquinone	Adriamycin, Mitomycin C
Nitroso	denitrosation	CCNU (1-(2-chloroethyl)-nitrosourea)
Dehalogenation	$R-X \longrightarrow R^\bullet + X^-$ (X = halogen substituent)	Halothane Chloramphenicol

reductive drug metabolism is not as developed as that for oxidation reactions, some reductions have been relatively well characterised. For example, tertiary amine oxides are extensively reduced by a cytochrome P450-dependent mechanism whereby amine metabolite formation is catalysed by the sequential two-electron reduction of the haemoprotein in a similar manner to the mixed-function amine oxidase described above. In addition, hydroxylamine reduction is catalysed by two separate enzyme systems. One involves cytochrome P450 and the other involves an NADH H$^+$-dependent flavoprotein (F_p) enzyme system:

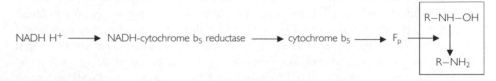

In this latter system, NADH H$^+$ serves as the preferred source of the necessary reducing equivalents which are then transferred by the cytochrome b$_5$ system to a terminal flavoprotein (F_p). This latter flavoprotein has been partially characterised from liver microsomes and actively catalyses the reduction of hydroxylamines, although the precise substrate specificity, and hence overall contribution to drug metabolism, still remains to be clarified. Similarly, although nitro- and azo-reduction pathways have been known for many years, a full understanding of the enzymes involved is far from complete. For example, the reduction of azo compounds like amaranth and other food colourants/dyes is catalysed by several enzyme systems including cytosolic DT-diaphorase, NADPH-cytochrome P450 reductase and cytochrome P450, the latter two enzymes either acting in concert or separately in catalysing azo reduction, depending on the specific substrate in question.

From the above discussion of the metabolism of amine-containing drugs, it is clear that metabolic oxidation/reduction cycling of drugs may occur. This represents an interesting concept in drug biotransformation reactions as the balance between oxidative and reductive pathways can be important in determining both the overall pharmacological and toxicological profile of the drug. For example, many drugs are active *per se*, whereas others require metabolic activation to express their toxicity, as is seen with many *N*-oxidised metabolites of drugs and xenobiotics.

Many anticancer drugs such as adriamycin and mitomycin C undergo reductive metabolism of their quinone moiety, a metabolic pathway that is a prerequisite for the anti-tumour properties of this class of drug. As shown in Figure 2.15, the quinone undergoes a one-electron reduction reaction catalysed by the microsomal flavoprotein NADPH-cytochrome P450 reductase (acting alone), resulting in the formation of the semi-quinone free radical species. This semi-quinone metabolite is unstable in the presence of oxygen and is rapidly re-oxidised to re-form the parent quinone and the superoxide anion radical. This latter cytotoxic reduction product is central to the mode of action of these anticancer drugs and is involved in binding to nucleic acids, DNA strand breakage and oxygen-dependent cytotoxicity. In addition, the anticancer quinone drugs are also metabolised by other

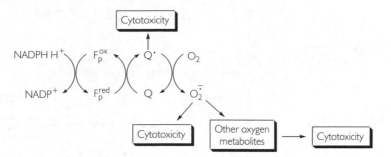

Figure 2.15 Role of NADPH-cytochrome P450 reductase in the metabolic activation of quinone anticancer drugs. Abbreviations used: F_p^{ox}, F_p^{red}, oxidised and reduced forms of NADPH-cytochrome P450 reductase, respectively; Q and Q', quinone and semi-quinone forms of the drug, respectively.

enzymes such as cytosolic DT-diaphorase, mitochondrial NADH dehydrogenase and xanthine oxidase, although the relative contributions made by these enzymes still remains to be clarified. Furthermore, it has recently been shown that NADPH-cytochrome P450 reductase is also responsible for the reductive denitrosation of the nitrosourea anticancer drugs such as CCNU (lomustine). This reductive pathway results in the formation of nitric oxide and the inactive, denitrosated parent urea and therefore represents a pharmacological deactivation pathway.

The above two examples highlight the versatility of the NADPH-cytochrome P450 reductase enzyme. In addition to functioning as an intrinsic component of the MFO system, this flavoprotein can independently catalyse the NADPH-dependent, one-electron reduction of quinones and nitrosoureas, thus utilising exogenous drugs as electron acceptors instead of the physiological acceptor, cytochrome P450.

Halothane is a volatile anaesthetic and this halogenated hydrocarbon is metabolised by both oxidative and reductive pathways in the liver. Whereas oxidative metabolism of halothane by the MFO system is generally considered to be a detoxication pathway, reductive metabolism of this anaesthetic has been implicated in the well-documented toxicity of this drug. As shown in Figure 2.16(a), halothane is reductively metabolised by two successive dehalogenation reactions (debromination and defluorination), metabolic pathways that are stimulated by enzyme induction with phenobarbital, thus implicating a role for the MFO system in these biotransformation processes. Further induction and inhibition studies point to a central role for cytochrome P450 in the reductive dehalogenation of halothane and the proposed participation of this haemoprotein is shown in Figure 2.16(b). This proposed mechanism has many features in common with the previously described MFO reaction of cytochrome P450 in that the scheme proposes substrate binding and two one-electron reduction steps (perhaps involving cytochrome b_5). However, the reaction mechanisms diverge in that, during the *anaerobic* reduction of halothane, no oxygen is present and hence the reducing equivalents are not used to activate molecular oxygen, but rather are contributory

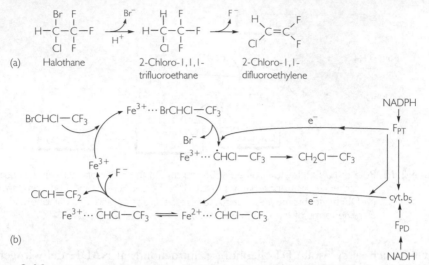

Figure 2.16 Reductive dehalogenation of halothane. (a) Halothane metabolism forming 2-chloro-1,1,1-trifluoroethane and 2-chloro-1,1-difluoroethylene. (b) Proposed reaction scheme for cytochrome P450 in the dehalogenation of halothane. Abbreviations used: Fe^{3+}, Fe^{2+}, the oxidised and reduced haem of P450, respectively; F_{PT}, NADPH-cytochrome P450 reductase; cyt b_5, cytochrome b_5, F_{PD}, NADH-cytochrome b_5 reductase.

to the formation of the radical and carbanion complexes of halothane, themselves the probable precursors of the dehalogenated metabolites. This reaction scheme may be superficially surprising in light of the high affinity of cytochrome P450 for oxygen and it may be predicted that oxygen would actively compete for the available reducing equivalents. However, certain cells have a very low oxygen tension, particularly in the centre of liver lobules and under these almost anaerobic conditions it is highly plausible that cytochrome P450 would function in a reductive mode, as described above. Accordingly, the prevailing tissue oxygen tension may very well be an important determinant of whether oxidative or reductive metabolism occurs.

2.6 EPOXIDE HYDROLASE

Among the many reactions catalysed by the microsomal MFO system is the oxidation of a number of olefins and aromatic compounds forming epoxide (alternatively called oxirane) metabolites, i.e. oxygen is inserted across a carbon–carbon double bond. These epoxides are formed as metabolites of drugs such as carbamazepine, cyproheptadine and protriptyline and other xenobiotics including environmental pollutants of the polycyclic aromatic (PAH) class of compounds. The epoxides thus formed have several biological fates, including direct excretion *in vivo*, non-enzymatic rearrangement forming phenols, irreversible binding to cellular nucleic acids and proteins, conjugation with glutathione, further oxidation

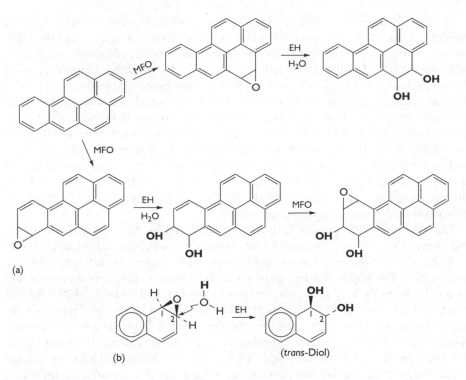

Figure 2.17 Epoxide formation and subsequent metabolism by epoxide hydrolase. (a) Scheme for the metabolism of the polycyclic aromatic hydrocarbon, benzo[*a*]pyrene (an air-borne environmental pollutant), resulting in the formation of epoxides, diols and diol-epoxides. (b) Stereospecific hydration of 1,2-naphthalene epoxide by epoxide hydrolase. Abbreviations used: MFO, mixed-function oxidase; EH, epoxide hydrolase.

to diol-epoxides or subject to enzymatic hydration to dihydrodiol metabolites, the latter being catalysed by a family of enzymes called the epoxide hydrolases. As shown in Figure 2.17(a), epoxidation can occur at various sites within the same molecule and subsequent epoxide ring opening by epoxide hydrolase leads to the formation of both diol and diol-epoxide metabolites.

Epoxides are chemically reactive, electrophilic species and epoxide hydrolase (sometimes called epoxide hydratase) catalyses the nucleophilic attack of a water molecule on one of the two electron-deficient carbon atoms of the epoxide ring. As shown in Figure 2.17(b), hydration of certain epoxide substrates can be highly stereoselective with respect to product formation, resulting in the predominant formation of the *trans* diol isomer of naphthalene. However, the degree of stereospecificity varies from one substrate to another and is governed by both steric and electronic characteristics of the substrate itself. In addition, it appears that the hydration reaction is also regioselective in that the less sterically hindered carbon atom in the 2-position of naphthalene (Figure 2.17(b)) incorporates water-derived oxygen more readily than the 1-position.

Epoxide hydrolase is widely distributed throughout the animal kingdom, including man. In the rat, it occurs in almost every tissue examined, with the highest concentrations being found in the liver and smaller, although significant, amounts expressed in the testes, kidney, lung and adrenal gland. Hepatic epoxide hydrolase has been found to be non-uniformly distributed across the liver lobule. Similar amounts are present in mid-zonal and periportal hepatocytes with significantly more enzyme present in centrilobular hepatocytes in uninduced rat liver, a distribution that accords with the distribution of most cytochromes P450. Thus, centrilobular hepatocytes appear to have the greatest capacity for both generating and hydrating epoxides. In the liver, epoxide hydrolase occurs predominantly in the endoplasmic reticulum and recent studies have indicated the enzyme to be present in nuclear membranes and the cytosol of the hepatocyte, but absent in peroxisomes, lysosomes and mitochondria.

The expression of epoxide hydrolase is increased by most of the xenobiotic inducers of the MFO system (see Chapter 3) and there is substantial evidence to suggest that the enzyme exists in multiple forms, with somewhat different substrate specificities. The highly purified enzymes derived from experimental animals and man exhibit monomeric molecular weights in the range of 48 000–54 000 daltons and UV/visible spectral analysis indicates the lack of both haem and flavin chromophore prosthetic groups. It is of interest that human liver microsomes contain relatively high levels of epoxide hydrolase activity and the enzyme from this source has been purified and characterised. There is a substantial variation in enzyme expression within the human population, suggesting that xenobiotic induction observed in experimental animals is also of relevance to man. Furthermore, human liver contains at least four forms of epoxide hydrolase.

In addition to metabolising the epoxides of drugs and xenobiotics, it should be remembered that epoxide hydrolase also catalyses the hydration of endogenous epoxides. These include $16\alpha,17\alpha$-epoxyandrosten-3-one (androstene oxide) and $16\alpha,17\alpha$-epoxyestratrienol (estroxide) at much higher rates than for xenobiotic epoxides, suggesting a substantial role for this enzyme in endogenous metabolic pathways.

Much attention has focused on epoxide hydrolase, primarily because of the role played by the enzyme in the formation of chemical carcinogens from otherwise innocuous xenobiotics (see Chapter 6 for a fuller discussion of this phenomenon).

2.7 GLUCURONIDE CONJUGATION REACTIONS

As discussed previously, phase 1 drug metabolism pathways represent a functionalisation reaction, in that the drug is chemically primed to facilitate subsequent conjugation reactions (phase 2) with endogenous compounds, thus enhancing their susceptibility to be excreted. One of the most important phase 2 conjugation reactions is that of conjugation with glucuronic acid, and many drugs are metabolised by this pathway. As shown in Table 2.8, many functional groups have the potential to be glucuronidated and it should be emphasised that the versatility of this reaction dictates that certain drugs can be directly conjugated with glucuronic

Table 2.8 Types of functional groups undergoing conjugation reactions with glucuronic acid

Functional group	Type	Example
Hydroxyl	Primary, secondary and tertiary, alcohols, phenols, hydroxylamines	Indomethacin, Paracetamol, 4-Hydroxy-coumarin, Aspirin, Chloromphen, Morphine
Carboxyl	Aromatic, arylalkyl	Nicotinic acid, Aminosalicylic acid, Clofibrate
Amino	Aromatic amines, sulfonamides, aliphatic tertiary amines	Meprobamate Dapsone Sulfafurazole
Sulfhydryl	Thiols, dithioic acids	2-Mercapto-benzothiazole

acid (providing they already possess a pre-existing functional group for conjugation), thus bypassing the usual requirement for phase 1 metabolism. In a similar manner to the MFO enzymes, many endogenous compounds serve as substrates for the glucuronidation reaction and include bilirubin, several steroid hormones, thyroxine, triiodothyronine and catechols derived from catecholamine metabolism. This observation raises the intriguing question of whether glucuronidation of drugs represents a late development by the organism and that the 'natural' role of this pathway is for endogenous compounds.

The enzymatic reaction mechanism for glucuronide formation and the fate of the conjugates is shown in Figure 2.18. The early stages of this reaction are involved in glycogen synthesis through the common intermediate of UDP-glucose and again highlights the intimate relationship between drug metabolism reactions and endogenous metabolic pathways. The readily available UDP-glucose may well explain the major role played by glucuronidation in drug metabolism. The enzyme that directly catalyses the conjugation of drugs with glucuronic acid is UDP-glucuronosyl transferase (alternatively known as glucuronyl transferase and abbreviated to UGT hereafter). It should be noted that the C-1 atom of glucuronic acid in UDP-glucuronic acid is in the α-configuration, and during transfer to an acceptor drug substrate inversion occurs resulting in the formation of the β-configuration. The resulting drug–glucuronide conjugate is then excreted in either the urine or faeces (Figure 2.18) and the molecular weight of the conjugate is a critical determinant in dictating the specific route of excretion. For example, glucuronide conjugates of molecular weight greater than approximately 400 daltons are excreted predominantly in the bile (i.e. drugs with molecular weights greater than approximately 200 daltons), whereas lower molecular weight conjugates primarily undergo urinary excretion. Thus high molecular weight drugs such as morphine, chloramphenicol and glutethimide, and glucuronide conjugates of both endogenous and exogenous steroids, are excreted in the bile and hence into

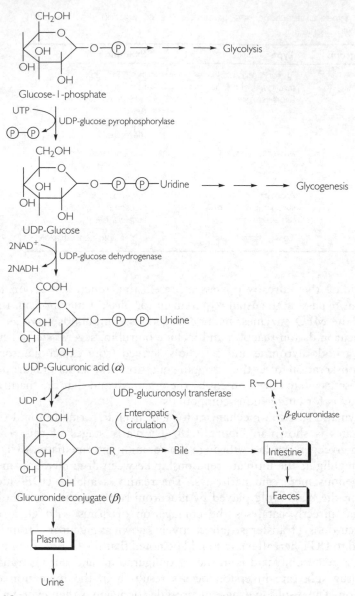

Figure 2.18 Formation of glucuronide conjugates and their biological fates. From Bowman and Rand (1980) *Textbook of Pharmacology*, 2nd edn, Blackwell Science.

the intestine. However, the intestine contains significant amounts of the enzyme β-glucuronidase (mainly in the gut flora), an enzyme that catalyses the hydrolysis of the glucuronide conjugate, resulting in the re-formation of the free drug, which may then be reabsorbed from the intestine, transported to the liver and then undergoes re-conjugation and re-excretion (Figure 2.19). This loop is called the enterohepatic circulation and may make a contribution to prolonging the half-life of the

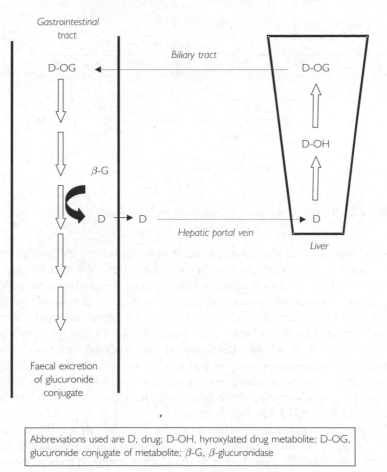

Gastrointestinal tract

Biliary tract

D-OG

D-OG

β-G

D-OH

D → D

Hepatic portal vein

D

Liver

Faecal excretion
of glucuronide
conjugate

Abbreviations used are D, drug; D-OH, hyroxylated drug metabolite; D-OG, glucuronide conjugate of metabolite; β-G, β-glucuronidase

Figure 2.19 The enterohepatic circulation of drugs and xenobiotics.

drug in the body, with the obvious result of potentiating the pharmacological action of the drug, providing that sufficiently high blood levels of the drug are achieved.

UGT is found in almost all mammalian species, with the notable exceptions of the cat and a mutant strain of rat (the Gunn rat). Cats have lost the UGT1A6 gene (via a mutation in exon 1), but express other UGT forms and are particularly sensitive to the pharmacological actions of morphine, an observation that is partially rationalised by the fact that the major route of morphine metabolism is normally by glucuronidation (via UGT1A6). The Gunn rat is an interesting example of enzyme deficiency in that this strain is completely incapable of forming glucuronide conjugates of bilirubin, whereas UGT activity towards most other substrates is apparently normal. The reason for this low transferase activity towards bilirubin is now becoming clearer as it has recently been reported that the Gunn rat has a − 1 frameshift mutation in exon 1 as determined by isolation and

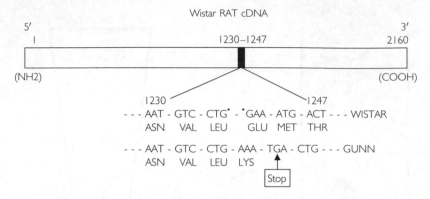

Figure 2.20 Frameshift mutation in the Gunn rat UDP-glucuronosyl transferase gene.

sequence comparison of the genes in the Wistar rat (wild type, normal activity) and the Gunn rat deficient. As shown in Figure 2.20, the crucial region is at nucleotide 1239 where a G residue is missing, thus generating a new TGA stop codon. Thus a truncated version of the transferase is generated by this new stop codon and the enzyme is missing the last 115 amino acids of the carboxyl terminus compared to the Wistar rat enzyme. This new carboxyl terminal in the Gunn rat has no hydrophobic character, is not inserted into the microsomal membrane and the truncated enzyme is degraded/secreted in the Golgi apparatus. It is instructive to note that this mutation occurs in exon 1 (an exon common to the whole UGT1 sub-family, see below) and therefore the Gunn rat does not express any of the UGT1 sub-family members.

UGT is present in many tissues, mostly in the liver, but also in the kidney, small intestine, lung, skin, adrenals and spleen. The enzyme is membrane bound in the endoplasmic reticulum and is therefore ideally positioned to glucuronidate the products of the MFO reaction. The enzyme has no prosthetic group and the monomeric molecular weight of homogeneous enzyme preparations varies from approximately 50 000–60 000 daltons. The catalytic activity of UGT is substantially influenced by the presence of lipids, although the specific mode of lipid action has not been elucidated. An interesting feature of UGT activity is that the membrane-bound enzyme exhibits 'latency', i.e. full enzyme activity is only observed in the presence of membrane perturbants such as detergents, and may be related to a barrier for the UDPGA transporter. The physiological and pharmacological significance (if any) of this enzyme latency has not been fully elucidated to date.

2.7.1 Multiple forms and nomenclature

The fact that UGT metabolises a broad range of structurally diverse endogenous and exogenous compounds led to the early belief that the enzyme exists in multiple forms. Based on the purification and characterisation of different, catalytically competent enzymes from various tissue sources and from molecular cloning, DNA sequencing and cDNA expression systems, it has now been firmly established that

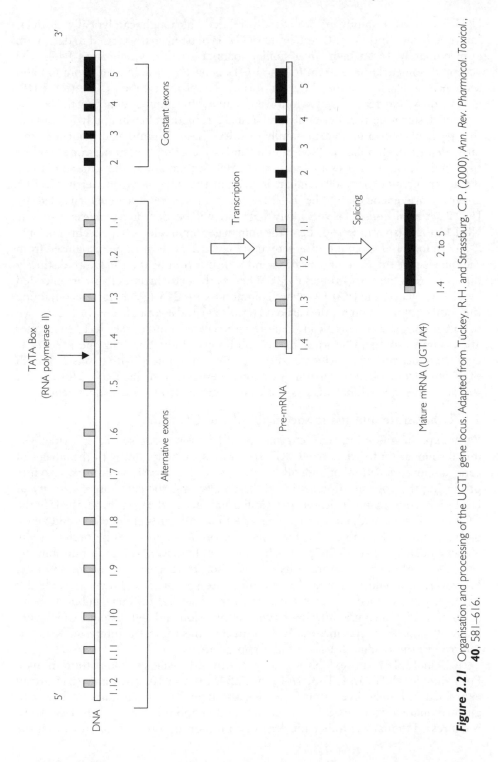

Figure 2.21 Organisation and processing of the UGT1 gene locus. Adapted from Tuckey, R.H. and Strassburg, C.P. (2000), *Ann. Rev. Pharmacol. Toxicol.*, **40**, 581–616.

UGT exists as a family of structurally related, although catalytically distinct, multiple forms, and over 50 vertebrate UGTs have been characterised to date, with approximately 16 in man. In a similar manner to the cytochromes P450, the accepted nomenclature system for the UGTs is based on divergent evolution and sequence similarity of the different forms. The root symbol UGT (for UDP-glucuronosyltransferase) is used followed by an Arabic number denoting the family, a letter designating the sub-family and a final Arabic number uniquely identifying that particular form in that sub-family (e.g. UGT1A4). Amino acid sequence simi-larity defines the families and sub-families and two enzymes are in the same family if their amino acid sequences are greater than 50% similar and in the same sub-family if they are greater than 60% similar. In man, at the time of writing, eight UGT1A enzymes are encoded by the UGT1A locus and seven proteins encoded by UGT2 genes, although it is very likely that more will be identified in due course. The UGT1A locus (spanning 160 kbp in the human genome) is localised on chromosome 2-q37 in man and is organised as shown in Figure 2.21. It must be recognised from the outset that the gene organisation and transcription of the UGTs are distinctly different from the cytochromes P450. Whereas the cytochromes P450 are encoded by distinct genes, the UGT1As share common exons 2–5 (gene regions containing the coding information for the carboxyl terminus) and a variable exon 1 (12 known to date, Figure 2.21). This means that the carboxyl terminus of the UGT1A enzymes are common to the 12 forms in this sub-family. Individual enzyme identity is conferred, depending on which of the 12 exon 1s are spliced with exons 2–5, each of which is controlled by separate promoter elements 5' to the exon. However, it should be recognised that UGT1s and UGT2s are coded for by distinct genes.

2.7.2 Substrate and tissue specificity of the UGTs

Early experiments using UGT enzymes purified from tissue sources provided the initial foundation for classifying UGT substrate specificity, but with the advent of gene cloning, isolation of individual cDNAs and expression of these enzymes producing the cognate proteins in cell-based systems, the substrate specificity of UGTs is becoming much clearer. In a similar manner to the cytochromes P450, the UGTs exhibit a broad, but overlapping, specificity towards endogenous and xeno-biotic compounds (Table 2.9). For example, opioids appear to be preferentially glucuronidated by UGT2B7, primary amines by UGT1A6 and bilirubin by UGT1A1, although in the majority of cases substrate specificity is not absolute. However, it should be noted that the substrate specificities shown in Table 2.9 have yet to be refined as they are compiled from several different publications in the literature, which use differing enzyme expression and cell systems, which very likely alter substrate specificities. With respect to this topic, the interested reader is referred to the reading list for a fuller appreciation.

UGT multiple forms exhibit a quite pronounced tissue-specific pattern in man. For example, UGTs 1A1, 1A3, 1A4, 1A6, 2B4, 2B7, 2B10, 2B11 and 2B15 are all expressed in human liver, thus providing the liver with a substantial capacity to glucuronidate a wide range of endogenous and xenobiotic compounds. UGT1A10 is expressed in many extrahepatic organs, an important observation in view of the

Table 2.9 Substrate specificities of UGTs

Substrate	UGT activity[a]									
	1A1	1A3	1A4	1A6	1A8	2A1	2B4	2B7	2B15	2B17
Simple phenols	1900	239	30	2400	5300	735	0.4	5	167	38
Bilirubin	400	0	2	0	0	nd	0	0	0	0
Carboxylic acids	0	121	0	nd	170	68	0	2	0	nd
Primary amines	1	84	540	10600	1800	22	nd	3	0	nd
Opioids	0	130	0	0	0	73	0	3462	0	nd

[a] Data are maximum specific enzyme activities (pmol/min/mg protein). nd, not determined. Adapted from Tukey and Strassburg (2000) *Ann. Rev. Pharmacol. Toxicol.* **40**, 581–616. Note that these substrate specificities have yet to be further refined (see text).

fact that this form exhibits one of the widest ranges of substrate specificities of known UGTs, ranging from small phenolic compounds to large steroids. In addition, UGT1A10 is expressed in all regions of the gastrointestinal tract, thus providing a first line of defence for the elimination of orally administered xenobiotics which have the capability to be directly glucuronidated.

2.7.3 UGT polymorphisms

Although several studies have implied an interindividual variation in the ability of man to glucuronidate drugs, the underlying reasons for this are not clear. It is possible that this phenomenon may be rationalised in part by genetic polymorphisms in the UGTs and it is instructive to note that patients suffering from hereditary hyperbilirubinaemia (clinically manifested by very high levels of unconjugated bilirubin and hence jaundice) have several different mutations in the UGT1 family genes. This gene locus encodes several UGTs capable of conjugating drugs and may therefore underpin interindividual variation in drug glucuronidation capacity in man, a hypothesis which remains to be confirmed. In contrast, the glucuronidation of bilirubin (catalysed by UGT1A1) exhibits a well-defined polymorphism as in hereditary hyperbilirubinaemia mentioned above. The molecular genetics of this group of diseases have been reasonably well characterised and are manifested in man as either Gilbert's disease (mild) or the Crigler–Najjar syndrome (severe), wherein different mutations (at least 33) in either the UGT1A1 promoter or coding regions have been identified. It appears that one single UGT1A1 mutation is sufficient to cause hyperbilirubinaemia.

2.8 GLUTATHIONE-*S*-TRANSFERASE

The glutathione-*S*-transferase family of enzymes are proteins which are widely distributed in the body, particularly in liver cytosol, and which catalyse the conjugation of a variety of compounds with the endogenous tripeptide glutathione (glutamylcysteinylglycine, abbreviated to GSH) as follows:

$$R-CH_2-X \xrightarrow[\text{GSH}]{\text{Glutathione-S-transferase}} R-CH_2-SG$$

Table 2.10 Role of glutathione-*S*-transferases in the conjugation and binding of endogenous and exogenous compounds

Binding function	Conjugation function
Bilirubin	Vitamin K$_3$
Oestradiol	Oestradiol-17β
Cortisol	Paracetamol
Testosterone	Sulfobromophthalein
Tetracycline	Parathion
Penicillin	Urethane
Ethacrynic acid	1-Chloro-2,4-dinitrobenzene

where $R-CH_2-X$ represents literally hundreds of electrophilic drugs and xenobiotics, and $R-CH_2-SG$ represents the glutathione adduct. In addition to their ability to catalyse the above conjugation reaction, certain glutathione-*S*-transferases have the ability to bind a variety of endogenous and exogenous substrates without metabolism. Examples of these two distinct roles of glutathione-*S*-transferase are given in Table 2.10. It should be emphasised that glutathione conjugation is possible with either unchanged drugs or their electrophilic metabolites, the only apparent chemical prerequisite being the presence of a suitably electrophilic centre enabling reactivity with the nucleophilic glutathione. In this respect, glutathione conjugation significantly differs from both glucuronide and sulfate conjugation in that, in the latter two reactions, both the glucuronide and sulfate moieties must first be 'activated' in the form of UDP-glucuronic acid and 3'-phosphoadenosine-5'-phosphosulfate respectively, prior to conjugation. Such chemical reactivity of glutathione and electrophiles can, in some cases, allow the conjugation reaction to proceed non-enzymatically. As with the high molecular weight glucuronide conjugates, glutathione metabolites are infrequently removed from the body by urinary excretion and preferential elimination occurs in the bile.

Many glutathione conjugates are not excreted *per se* but rather undergo further enzymatic modification of the peptide moiety, resulting in the urinary or biliary excretion of cysteinyl-sulfur substituted *N*-acetylcysteines, more commonly referred to as mercapturic acids. As shown in Figure 2.22 for an arene oxide metabolite, mercapturic acid formation is initiated by glutathione conjugation, followed by removal of the glutamate moiety by glutathionase and subsequent removal of glycine by a peptidase enzyme, the latter two enzymes being present in the liver, gastrointestinal tract and kidney. In the final step, the amino group of cysteine is acetylated by a hepatic *N*-acetylase, resulting in the formation of the mercapturic acid derivative. This latter acetylation reaction is reversible and deacetylases can re-form the amino metabolite.

The cysteine conjugate of xenobiotics can undergo an alternative metabolic pathway by serving as a substrate for the cysteine conjugate β-lyase enzyme (see Chapter 1) which catalyses the following β-elimination reaction:

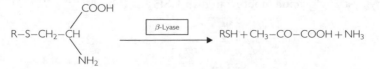

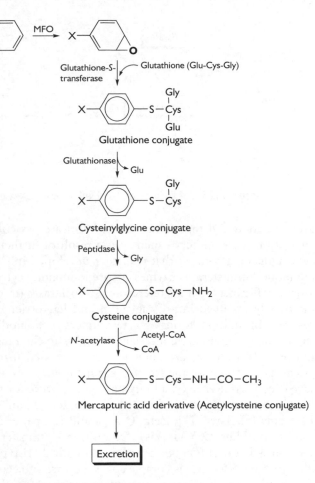

Figure 2.22 Role of glutathione in mercapturic acid biosynthesis.

The cysteine conjugate β-lyase enzymes occur in several tissues, including the gastrointestinal tract, liver and kidney, and the renal and hepatic forms have been the most extensively studied. All β-lyase enzymes studied to date contain pyridoxal phosphate, and, as such, the enzyme *additionally* functions as a transaminase and therefore exhibits a sophisticated level of regulation (Figure 2.23). The monomeric molecular weights of the β-lyases are around 48 000 daltons and the liver form is also known as kynureninase and the kidney form as glutamine transaminase K. It appears that multiple forms of cysteine conjugate β-lyase exist and certainly the liver and kidney forms are distinct proteins.

From the above discussion it is clear that glutathione conjugation serves as a protective mechanism whereby potentially toxic electrophilic metabolites are 'mopped up' either as glutathione conjugates or mercapturic acids. However, it is becoming increasingly recognised that glutathione conjugation is not exclusively a

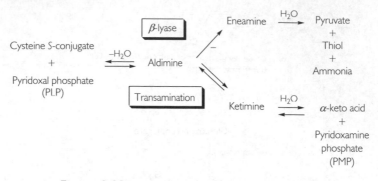

Figure 2.23 Dual activity of cysteine conjugate β-lyase.

detoxification reaction and that certain xenobiotics are toxicologically activated by this conjugation route, either as such or as a result of further processing of the glutathione conjugate, a concept that is further developed in Chapter 6.

The glutathione-S-transferase enzymes are predominantly cytosolic enzymes and are evolutionarily distinct from the microsomal transferases (termed MAPEG), the latter being mostly involved in prostaglandin and leukotriene metabolism. The transferases exist in multiple forms as heterodimers or homodimers of two sub-units, of approximate monomeric molecular weights in the range 20 000–25 000 daltons and over 20 isoforms are known to be expressed in man. The nomen-clature system has been confusing for this group of enzymes as several different systems have been used. Recently, a unifying nomenclature for the soluble human transferases has been suggested and classified into gene families (Alpha [A], Mu [M], Pi [P], Sigma [S], Theta [T], Zeta, Omega and Kappa) and reflect their sub-unit compositions. Thus GSTA1-1 is a glutathione-S-transferase (GST) of the Alpha class, consisting of a homodimer of two identical '1'-type sub-units.

Regulation of the GST genes is complex and they are subject to developmental control, display tissue-specific expression, are responsive to physiological stress, exhibit sex-specificity and are inducible by structurally diverse xenobiotics includ-ing butylated hydroxyanisole, ethoxyquin, oltipraz, coumarin, indole-3-carbinol, TCDD and polycyclic aromatic hydrocarbons. In the case of heterodimers, each sub-unit may be differently and independently regulated by transcriptional gene activation mechanisms. Several xenobiotic responsive elements for inducers are localised in GST promoters and other cellular transcription factors are recruited to facilitate the transcriptional activation of responsive GST genes.

GST polymorphisms are known to exist in several species (including man) and are subject to differential distribution between ethnic races. For example, two different mutations in the GSTM1 gene (termed GSTM1*0 and GSTM1*B) are present in Chinese (58%, 29%), English (52%, 16%) and Nigerian (22%, 6%) populations, respectively. Significantly, 90% of Polynesians have been reported to be null for the GSTM1 gene. In view of the fact that most GSTs protect against xenobiotic-induced toxicity, much effort is being expended in trying to associate the existence of nullifying GST mutations (particularly GSTM1) with susceptibility to disease, including chemically induced cancer. In particular, polymorph-isms in the GSTM1 gene has attracted especial attention as it detoxifies polycyclic aromatic hydrocarbons found in cigarette smoke and environmentally derived combustion products. To date, allelic variants have been identified in the GSTA2, GSTM1, GSTM3, GSTM4, GSTP1, GSTT1, GASTZ1MGST1, LTC4S and PLAP loci and the interested reader is referred to the reading list for further, specific information on GST polymorphisms.

2.9 SULFATE CONJUGATION

Many drugs are oxidised to a variety of phenols, alcohols or hydroxylamines that can then serve as excellent substrates for subsequent sulfate conjugation, forming the readily excretable sulfate esters. However, inorganic sulfate is relatively inert and must first be 'activated' by ATP as in the following reaction sequence:

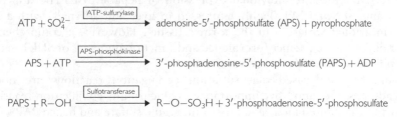

The key enzyme in this sequence is sulfotransferase and the mammalian sulfo-transferase enzymes (hereafter referred to as SULT) are soluble enzymes found in many tissues including liver, kidney, gut and platelets and which catalyse the sulfation of drugs such as paracetamol, isoprenaline and salicylamide and several endogenous compounds such as steroids, catecholamines and thyroid hormone. The SULTs exist in multiple enzyme forms and at least 45 SULTs have been identified in mammals with at least 11 genes in man, the latter being dispersed on five separate chromosomes. As we have seen before for the cytochromes P450 and UGTs, the mammalian SULTs are classified into gene families (SULTs 1–5), with families being differentiated from each other by having less than 45% amino acid sequence similarity to the other families. The families are further sub-divided into sub-families (45–60% similar) and individual genes being uniquely identified by an Arabic number (e.g. SULT1A1). Mammalian SULTs fall into the SULT1 and SULT2 families, a SULT 3 family has recently been identified in rabbits (catalysing sulfamate formation) and SULTs 4 and 5 have been recently identified in DNA sequence data bases, although the enzymes have not been characterised to date. A single member of the SULT6 family has been found in chickens. SULT1 has five sub-families (A–E) and SULT2 has 2 (A, B). As shown in Table 2.11, the SULTs catalyse the sulfation of a broad range of endogenous and xenobiotic compounds, with some forms exhibiting a relatively selective substrate selectivity whereas others are more promiscuous. The SULTs have a fairly wide tissue distribution, but the molecular mechanisms underpinning tissue-specific expression and gene regulation still remain to be clarified.

Table 2.11 Substrate specificity of SULTs

SULT	Substrates
SULT1As (not 1A3)	p-nitrophenol, α-naphthol
SULT1A3	Dopamine and other catecholamines
SULT1B1	Thyroid hormones
SULT1C1	N-hydroxy-2-acetylaminofluorene
SULT1D	5-HT, ecosanoids, dopamine, p-nitrophenol
SULT1Es	Endogenous and xenobiotic estrogens
SULT2As/2Bs	Steroids and xenobiotic alcohols
SULT3A1	Amine N-sulphation forming sulphamates

Phenotypic/allelic variations have been noted in man, including four allozymes of SULT1A1, a wide interindividual expression of hepatic SULT1B2 and three allelic variants of SULT2A1 (highly expressed in liver and adrenals, with a five-fold interindividual variation in the former tissue). However, a comprehensive understanding of the existence, prevalence and functional impact of SULT genetic polymorphisms still remains to be resolved.

It should be emphasised that sulfation conjugation reactions are not as widespread or as of quantitative importance as glucuronide conjugation reactions, due in part to the limited bioavailability of inorganic sulfate and hence PAPS. This is particularly true when a drug is actively metabolised to phenolic products or when high body burdens of phenolic drugs are reached (for example, in over-dosage), resulting in effective saturation of this metabolic pathway.

2.10 AMINO ACID CONJUGATION

Many classes of drugs including anti-inflammatories of the profen class, hypo-lipidaemics, diuretics and analgesic agents have a carboxylic acid as part of their structure and, as such, are susceptible to conjugation with endogenous amino acids prior to excretion. In a similar manner to both glucuronide and sulfate conjugation, amino acid conjugation of free carboxylic acid groups in drugs requires metabolic activation, according to the following scheme:

$$R-COOH + ATP \longrightarrow R-CO-AMP + H_2O$$

$$R-CO-AMP + CoASH \longrightarrow R\text{-}CO\text{-}SCoA + AMP$$

$$R-CO-SCoA + NH_2-R'-COOH \longrightarrow R-CONH-R'\text{-}COOH + CoASH$$

where R−COOH represents the drug, CoASH is coenzyme A and $NH_2-R'-$COOH is an endogenous amino acid. In this scheme, the inert carboxyl group is activated to its acyl coenzyme-A derivative prior to amide formation with the amino function of the donating amino acid. As shown in Table 2.12, this conjugation reaction occurs in many species, utilising a variety of amino acids and appears to be a complementary pathway to the glucuronidation of carboxyl groups.

Table 2.12 Amino acids utilised in the conjugation of carboxylic acids

Amino acid	Species	Acid
Glycine	Mammals, non-primate mammals	Aromatic, heterocyclic and acrylic acids, arylacetic acids
Glutamine	Primates, rat, rabbit, ferret	Arylacetic acids, 2-naphthylacetic acid
Taurine	Mammals, pigeon	Arylacetic acids
Ornithine	Birds	Aromatic and arylacetic acids
Glutamic acid	Fruit bats	Benzoic acid
Aspartic acid	Rat	o,p'-DDA
Alanine	Mouse, hamster	p,p'-DDA
Histidine	African bats	Benzoic acid

Derived from Caldwell, J. (1980) In: *Concepts in Drug Metabolism, Part A* (P. Jenner and B. Testa, eds), Marcel Dekker, New York, p 221.

This conjugation reaction occurs extensively in hepatic mitochondria and has been used to advantage in chemical tests of liver function. For example benzoic acid is conjugated with glycine, resulting in excretion of the benzyl glycine conjugate, sometimes referred to as hippuric acid. Under conditions of normal liver function, a specified amount of hippuric acid is excreted within a few hours after either oral administration or slow intravenous injection of a specific dose. In parenchymal liver disorders such as hepatitis or cirrhosis, the urinary output of hippuric acid is low (assuming normal renal function) and therefore constitutes a useful indicator of hepatic viability.

2.11 CONTROL AND INTERACTIONS OF DRUG METABOLISM PATHWAYS

From the previous chapter and the above discussion, it is clear that ingested drugs can be metabolised by a variety of chemical pathways, catalysed by different

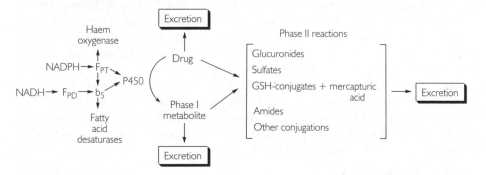

Figure 2.24 Drug metabolism pathways. Abbreviations used: F_{PT}, NADPH-cytochrome P450 reductase; F_{PD}, NADH-cytochrome b_5 reductase; P450, cytochrome P450; b_5, cytochrome b_5.

enzyme systems (Figure 2.24). As with most biotransformation pathways, drug metabolism reactions do not usually occur at random and specific biological control mechanisms are operative at several stages in the overall process. In addition, a particular drug metabolism pathway does not usually operate in isolation and the activity of one pathway can influence the activity in another. Furthermore, many drug biotransformation pathways are intimately related to endogenous metabolic pathways sharing both the same source of co-factors, co-substrates, prosthetic groups and even enzyme systems, thereby imposing an additional level of control on drug metabolism. The above concepts will be developed in this section, and where possible, specific examples will be given.

2.11.1 Substrate and oxygen availability

The majority of drugs are lipophilic in nature and therefore metabolism represents an efficient means of clearing the drug from the body. If metabolism is a prominent feature of clearance, then the 'bioavailability' of the drug assumes an important role in that the more readily accessible the drug is to the drug metabolising enzymes, then the greater will be its metabolism. Accordingly, the physicochemical properties of the drug, such as degree of ionisation or lipophilicity, are important in dictating the absorption of the drug and access to the membrane-bound or soluble drug-metabolising enzymes. As most of the phase 1 oxidation enzymes are located in the lipid-rich, and therefore lipophilic, membrane of the hepatic endoplasmic reticulum, it then follows that a substantial degree of drug lipophilicity is required to ensure adequate substrate availability. Many studies have shown that this is indeed the case and significant correlations have been repeatedly found between the lipid–water partition coefficient of drugs and their extent of binding to and metabolism by the phase 1 enzymes in general, and cytochrome P450 in particular. Therefore, the physicochemical nature of the drug itself is an important determinant of drug availability and hence potential to be metabolised.

As discussed previously, molecular oxygen is an essential requirement for cytochrome P450-dependent monooxygenation of drugs. In most body tissues, oxygen is freely available and in sufficiently high concentrations to ensure adequate drug oxidation. However, tissue concentrations of oxygen may well be very low under certain pathophysiological conditions and in the relatively hypoxic centre of the liver mass, thus placing a possible constraint, and therefore control, on drug oxidation. The availability of oxygen is an important determinant of the route or pathway of drug metabolism. For example, halothane is metabolised by both oxidative and reductive anaerobic pathways (see above), yielding metabolites that are quite different from each other and, more importantly, these metabolites have been postulated to have different toxicities. Although our understanding of the role of tissue levels of oxygen in drug metabolism is still in its infancy, it remains an area of fundamental importance.

2.11.2 NADPH supply

NADPH is an obligatory requirement for cytochrome P450-dependent drug oxidation, and therefore the availability of this reduced pyridine nucleotide is an

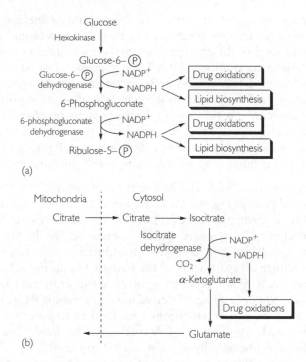

Figure 2.25 Biosynthesis of NADPH utilised in drug oxidation. (a) Pentose phosphate pathway. (b) NADPH-linked isocitrate dehydrogenase.

important control mechanism in drug metabolism. As shown in Figure 2.25, hepatic NADPH is derived from two sources, the major pathway being the pentose phosphate pathway (sometimes referred to as the hexose monophosphate shunt), further augmented by reducing equivalents derived from the mitochondrial translocation of NADPH. In addition to supplying the necessary reducing equivalents for drug oxidations, NADPH is required in endogenous biosynthetic pathways including fatty acid biosynthesis. For example, during the biosynthesis of palmitic acid starting from acetyl-CoA, 14 moles of NADPH are consumed per mole of palmitic acid formed, thus placing a substantial demand on the availability of cellular NADPH during active lipid biosynthesis. In addition, the availability of NADPH for drug oxidation is critically influenced by the cellular $NADP^+/NADPH$ ratio, which in turn is linked to the activity of the $NADP^+$- linked dehydrogenases such as isocitrate dehydrogenase and glucose-6-phosphate dehydrogenase. Accordingly, the availability of NADPH for drug oxidation is substantially influenced by prevailing metabolic conditions forming a coupled, interactive system and therefore constitutes a control point in drug oxidation.

2.11.3 Synthesis and degradation of cytochrome P450

In any enzyme-catalysed reaction, the absolute amount of active enzyme contributes to the overall reaction; thus the concentration or amount of the drug metabolising enzymes are clearly important. As the amount of enzyme present is a dynamic balance between enzyme synthesis and enzyme degradation, factors that alter the steady-state level of the enzymes then make a significant contribution to the regulation of drug metabolism. Of all the enzymes responsible for drug metabolism, cytochrome P450 has been the most intensively studied and the biogenesis and catabolism of this haemoprotein will now be considered, with particular emphasis placed on the role of haemoprotein turnover as a control mechanism in drug oxidation. It must be emphasised that the following concepts are also applicable to the regulation of the other drug metabolising enzymes, and that cytochrome P450 is only being used here as a well-documented example.

(a) *Synthesis of cytochrome P450.* The holoenzyme of cytochrome P450 consists of both haem and protein moieties, and are therefore subject to different control mechanisms in their biosynthesis, both of which contribute to the final, steady-state level of the enzyme. As shown in Figure 2.26, the biosynthesis of intact cytochrome P450 is a complex, coordinated process and involves different sub-cellular compartments of the hepatocyte during assembly of the intact holoenzyme. A major point of control is the utilisation of the haem prosthetic group. Not only is haem inserted into cytochrome P450, but it is also inserted into mitochondrial cytochromes and other hepatic haemoproteins such as catalase and cytochrome b_5. Accordingly, the total hepatic demand for haem is dictated not only by cytochrome P450 but also by other cellular haemoproteins, again illustrating the interrelationship between drug oxidation

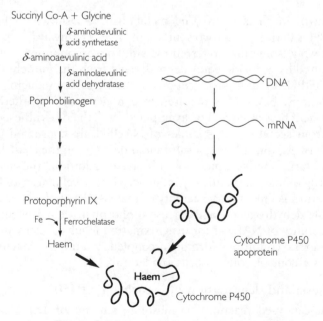

Figure 2.26 Biosynthesis of cytochrome P450.

and normal cellular processes. In addition, many drugs and chemicals have the ability to influence haem biosynthesis by either inducing the enzyme delta-aminolaevulinic acid synthetase, the rate-limiting step in haem biosynthesis, or by causing a depletion of existing free haem. This latter point is noteworthy because δ-aminolaevulinic acid synthetase is subjected to negative feedback inhibition by haem. Therefore certain drugs that initiate haem depletion can cause a 'rebound' effect in haem synthesis, resulting in acute attacks of porphyria in genetically predisposed individuals

Synthesis of the apoprotein moiety of cytochrome P450 is also subjected to control by the ability of drugs (such as the barbiturates, amongst others) to induce protein synthesis. Although drug induction of cytochrome P450 is considered in more detail in Chapter 3, it is relevant to point out that not only is cytochrome P450 induced by drugs, but different multiple forms are induced by different drugs. These cytochrome P450 enzymes exhibit substantial differences in their respective abilities to catalyse the oxidation of structurally diverse drugs, and it is then quite clear that the isoform complement of individual haemoproteins is an important determinant of the ability of the liver to metabolise a specific drug. In view of the common occurrence of polypharmacy, where patients are exposed to more than one drug (one of which may be an enzyme inducer), this 'drug-induced control mechanism' has significant ramifications in both clinical pharmacology and toxicology (see Chapters 6 and 7).

(b) *Degradation of cytochrome P450.* The major pathway of haem degradation involves an enzyme termed haem oxygenase, resulting in the eventual formation of bile pigments such as bilirubin. The complete microsomal haem oxygenase system requires both the haem oxygenase protein and the flavoprotein, NADPH-cytochrome P450 reductase. The participation of this latter flavoprotein is interesting in that NADPH-cytochrome P450 reductase is also a necessary component of the cytochrome P450-dependent drug oxidation system, as discussed previously. Therefore, during the normal course of drug oxidation, the flow of reducing equivalents through the reductase is not exclusively channelled to cytochrome P450, and during periods of active hepatic haem oxidation, there is competition exerted on the oxidation reaction by haem oxygenase activity, thus exerting another level of control on drug oxidation. In addition, many drugs and chemicals, especially those with an olefinic moiety, have the ability to covalently bind to and inactivate the haem group of cytochrome P450. This would then constitute another control mechanism whereby cytochrome P450 activity (and hence certain drug oxidation reactions) is substantially inhibited by prior or concomitant exposure to this class of drug.

2.11.4 Control of drug metabolism by endogenous co-substrates

As shown in Table 2.13, many of the enzymes of drug metabolism also catalyse the metabolism of a plethora of endogenous substrates. Some of these enzymes are relatively specific for the metabolism of endogenous substrates such as steroids

Table 2.13 Endogenous co-substrates of the drug metabolising enzymes

Cytochrome P450	Glucuronosyl transferase	Glutathione transferase
Fatty acids	Bilirubin	Bilirubin
Leukotrienes	Serotonin	Cortisol
Prostaglandins	Testosterone	Testosterone
Steroids		Glutathione
Cholesterol		Leukotrienes
Vitamin D_3		
Thyroxine		

(Figure 2.27), whereas others, such as hepatic cytochrome P450, are less specialised and catalyse steroid, fatty acid and prostaglandin hydroxylation in addition to drug oxidation. For this latter type of drug metabolising enzyme, there is therefore a competition for available enzyme between the drug and the endogenous substrate. Many factors are important in determining which substrate will be preferentially metabolised, including the tissue levels, the effective local concentration at the active site and the relative affinities of the competing substrates for the enzyme in question. As many endogenous substrates are in a constant state of flux due to synthesis, utilisation and degradation reactions, it is obvious that a precise analysis of the role of the endogenous co-substrates as competitors for the enzyme systems *in vivo* is difficult. Nevertheless, it is absolutely clear that competition does occur *in vitro* and therefore represents another mechanism whereby drug metabolism is subjected to a degree of control.

2.11.5 Participation of cytochrome b_5

As indicated earlier, the role of cytochrome b_5 in drug oxidation reactions is variable, as no uniform effect has been observed. For example, cytochrome b_5 has been reported to either stimulate, inhibit, have no effect or even be an obligatory

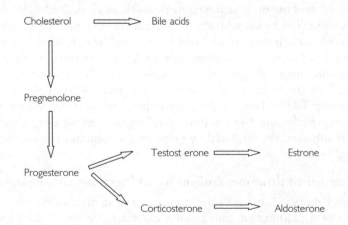

Figure 2.27 Importance of cytochrome P450 and steroid hydroxylation in liver and adrenal cortex.

component of cytochrome P450-dependent oxidation reactions, depending on both the nature of the drug undergoing metabolism and the particular form of cytochrome P450 under consideration. In those reactions that depend on cytochrome b_5, electron flow occurs as

NADH $\longrightarrow$ NADH-cytochrome b_5 reductase $\longrightarrow$ cytochrome b_5 $\longrightarrow$ cytochrome P450

It should be noted that cytochrome b_5 is also reduced by NADPH-cytochrome P450 reductase, thereby placing another 'drain' on the reducing equivalents of this flavoprotein. The main endogenous biological function of hepatic microsomal cytochrome b_5 is to participate in the desaturation of long-chain, fatty acid acyl-CoA derivatives, by providing reducing equivalents for the terminal desaturase enzymes. The desaturation of fatty acids in the endoplasmic reticulum is an active process and includes the $\Delta 5$-, $\Delta 6$- and $\Delta 9$-desaturases, and therefore constitutes a potent drain on cytochrome b_5-mediated reducing equivalents, and consequently significantly influences those drug oxidation reactions mediated by cytochrome b_5. In addition, unlike cytochrome P450, cytochrome b_5 is relatively insensitive to induction by exogenous drugs and chemicals. In uninduced liver microsomes, the molar ratio of cytochrome P450 : cytochrome b_5 is approximately 2 : 1 and during induction this can increase to around 6 : 1 or sometimes higher. Therefore the molecular association between these two haemoproteins is almost certainly influenced by induction and may then significantly alter both quantitative and qualitative aspects of drug metabolism.

2.11.6 Glucuronidation

As indicated in Figure 2.18, the conjugation of drugs and their metabolites with glucuronic acid is intimately related to carbohydrate metabolism, via UDP-glucuronic acid (UDPGA), the donor of the glucuronide moiety. The synthesis of UDPGA is not the sole metabolic pathway for glucose-1-phosphate and UDP-glucose and these two intermediates are important in both glycolysis and glyco-genesis pathways. From the viewpoint that glucuronidation is both an extensive and a not readily saturable reaction, it would appear that, under normal metabolic conditions, the supply of UDPGA is not rate-limiting in conjugation reactions. However, under conditions of excessive utilisation of carbohydrate or glycogen-esis, the flux of UDPGA through glucuronidation-based mechanisms is impaired, again illustrating the interaction of drug metabolism with normal metabolic processes. In addition, like cytochrome P450, the UDP-glucuronosyltransferases are subjected to induction by clinically used drugs and are important in the metab-olism of endogenous compounds. Therefore the concepts discussed for cyto-chrome P450 are equally applicable to the UDP-glucuronosyltransferases leading to altered substrate specificity after induction and subjected to competition by endogenous substrates.

2.11.7 Cellular competition for glutathione

In addition to acting as a co-substrate for the glutathione-S-transferase-catalysed conjugation of electrophilic drugs and chemicals, glutathione has other cellular functions. Two molecules of glutathione are oxidised by the enzyme glutathione peroxidase (in the presence of an oxidised substrate such as lipid peroxides) forming the disulfide of glutathione. The glutathione disulfide may then in turn be reduced back to glutathione by the enzyme glutathione reductase, thus setting up a cycle of glutathione utilisation coupled to the detoxification of cellular peroxides. However, under conditions of oxidative stress when peroxide concentrations are high, the formation of glutathione disulfide exceeds the capacity of the reductase, and high glutathione disulfide levels build up, are removed from the hepatocyte and excreted in the bile. The net result of this process is to deplete the hepatocyte of glutathione and thereby reduce the availability of this co-substrate for the glutathione-S-transferase-catalysed conjugation of drugs.

Another major cellular utilisation of glutathione is in the biosynthesis of the leukotrienes, including leukotrienes LTD_4 and LTE_4. These leukotrienes are derived originally from arachidonic acid and condensation of leukotriene A_4 (an epoxide of arachidonic acid) with glutathione (catalysed by glutathione-S-transferase) results in formation of LTC_4 and subsequently LTD_4 and LTE_4. Accordingly, it is clear that, when there is a high cellular demand for glutathione in leukotriene biosynthesis, the available levels of glutathione for xenobiotic conjugation are decreased and may become limiting under certain pathophysiological situations.

In conclusion, it must be emphasised that both phase 1 and phase 2 drug metabolism pathways cannot be considered in isolation, but rather as part of a coupled, interactive system, interfacing directly with many endogenous metabolic pathways. As our knowledge of the pathways and enzymology of drug metabolism advances, then so too must our knowledge of their control and interaction with other enzyme systems.

FURTHER READING

Textbooks and symposia

Ioannides, C. (1996) *Cytochromes P450: Metabolic and Toxicological Aspects.* CRC Press, Boca Raton, FL.

Jefcoate, C.R. (1996) *Physiological Functions of Cytochrome P450 in Relation to Structure and Function. Advances in Molecular Biology Series*, Vol. 14. JAI Press, Greenwich, CN.

Kalow, W. (1992) *Pharmacogenetics of Drug Metabolism.* Pergamon, New York

Lewis, D.F.V. (1996) *Cytochromes P450: Structure, Function and Mechanism.* Taylor and Francis, London.

Testa, B. (1995) *The Metabolism of Drugs and Other Xenobiotics: Biochemistry of Redox Reactions.* Academic Press, London.

Woolf, T.F. (ed.) (1999) *Handbook of Drug Metabolism.* Marcel Dekker, New York, pp 131–145.

Reviews and original articles

Burchell, B. (1999) Transformation reactions. In: *Handbook of Drug Metabolism* (T.F. Woolf, ed.). Marcel Dekker, New York, pp 153–173.

Burchell, B. *et al* (1995) Minireview: specificity of human UDP-glucuronosyl transferases and xenobiotic glucuronidation. *Life Sci.* **57**, 1819–1831.

Cashman, J.R. *et al* (2000) Population-specific polymorphisms of the human FMO3 gene: significance for detoxication. *Drug Metab. Disp.* **28**, 169–173.

Clarke, S.E. (1998) *In vitro* assessment of human cytochrome P450. *Xenobiotica* **28**, 1167–1202.

Daly, A. (1999) Pharmacogenetics. In: *Handbook of Drug Metabolism* (T.F. Woolf, ed.). Marcel Dekker, New York, pp 175–202.

Grant, D.M. *et al.* (1992) Polymorphisms of N-acetyltransferase genes. *Xenobiotica* **22**, 1073–1081.

Guengerich, F.P. (1991) Reactions and significance of cytochrome P450 enzymes. *J. Biol. Chem.* **266**, 10 019–10 022.

Hayes, J.D. and Pulford, D.J. (1995) The glutathione S-transferase supergene family: regulation and the contribution of the isoenzymes to cancer chemoprotection and drug resistance. *Crit. Rev. Biochem. Mol. Biol.* **30**, 445–600.

Hayes, J.D. and Strange, R.C. (1995) Potential contribution of the glutathione S-transferase supergene family to resistance to oxidative stress. *Free Radical Res.* **22**, 193–207.

Hayes, J.D. and Strange, R.C. (2000) Glutathione S-transferase polymorphisms and their biological consequences. *Pharmacology* **6**, 154–166.

Honma, W. *et al.* (2001) Enzymatic characterisation and interspecies difference of phenol sulphotransferases, ST1A forms. *Drug Metab. Disp.* **29**, 274–281.

Hsieh, K.P. *et al.* (2001) Novel mutations of CYP3A4 in Chinese. *Drug Metab. Disp.* **29**, 268–273.

Levine, W.G. (1992) Azoreduction of drugs and other xenobiotics. In: *Progress in Drug Metabolism,* Vol. 13 (G.G. Gibson, ed.). Taylor and Francis, London, pp 179–216.

MacKenzie, P.I. *et al.* (1997) The UDP glucuronosyl transferase gene family: recommended nomenclature update based on evolutionary divergence. *Pharmacogenetics* **7**, 255–269.

Mannervik, B. *et al.* (1992) Nomenclature for human glutathione transferases. *Biochem. J.* **282**, 305–308.

Nagata, K. and Yamazoe, Y. (2000) Pharmacogenetics of sulfotransferase. *Ann. Rev. Pharmacol. Toxicol.* **40**, 159–176.

Nebert, D.W. *et al.* (1987/1989/1991/1993) The P450 gene superfamily: recommended nomenclature and updates. *DNA Cell Biol.* **6**, 1–11; **8**, 1–13; **10**, 1–14; **12**, 1–51.

Pelkonen, O. *et al.* (1998) Inhibition and induction of human cytochrome P450 (CYP) enzymes. *Xenobiotica* **28**, 1203–1253.

Rettie, A.E. and Fisher, M.B. (1999) Transformation enzymes: oxidative; non-P450. In: *Handbook of Drug Metabolism* (T.F. Woolf, ed.). Marcel Dekker, New York, pp 131–52.

Sata, F. *et al.* (2000) CYP3A4 allelic variants with amino acid substitutions in exons 7 and 12: evidence for an allelic variant with altered catalytic activity. *Pharmacogen. Genom.* **67**, 48–56.

Shimada, T. *et al.* (1994) Interindividual variations in human liver cytochrome P450 enzymes involved in the oxidation of drugs, carcinogens and toxic chemicals: studies with liver microsomes of 30 Japanese and 30 Caucasians. *J. Pharmacol. Exp. Ther.* **270**, 414–423.

Smith, D.A. *et al.* (1998) Human cytochromes P450: selectivity and measurement *in vivo. Xenobiotica* **28**, 1095–1128.

Smith, G. *et al.* (1998) Molecular genetics of the human cytochrome P450 monooxygenase superfamily. *Xenobiotica* **28**, 1129–1165.

Tanaka, E. (1999) Update: genetic polymorphisms of drug metabolising enzymes. *J. Clin. Pharm. Ther.* **24**, 323–329.

Tucker, G.T. *et al.* (1998) Determination of drug-metabolising enzyme activity *in vivo*: pharmacokinetic and statistical issues. *Xenobiotica* **28**, 1255–1273.

Tuckey, R.H. and Strassburg, C.P. (2000) Human UDP-glucuronosyltransferases: metabolism, expression and disease. *Ann. Rev. Pharmacol. Toxicol.* **40**, 581–616.

van der Weide, J. and Steijns, L.S. (1999) Cytochrome P450 enzyme system: genetic polymorphisms and impact on clinical pharmacology. *Ann. Clin. Biochem.* **36**, 722–729.

Web sites

- The UDP glycosyltransferase gene superfamily: recommended nomenclature update based on evolutionary divergence.
  http://www.unisa.edu.au/pharm_medsci/Gluc_trans/currnom.htm
- Human UGT activities and substrate specificities. http://www.AnnualReviews.org
- Directory of P450-containing systems (updates on P450 sequences).
  http://base.icgeb.trieste.it/p450/
- Cytochrome P450 databases, sequence alignments and nomenclature.
  http://drnelson.utmem.edu/CytochromeP450.html
- A resource for research on plant and insect cytochromes P450.
  http://ag.arizona.edu/p450/
- Cytochrome P450: a wealth of information on P450 structure (and related redox proteins), steroid ligands of P450s, selected references on P450-containing systems, families of structural domains of P450-containing systems, structural domains of P450-containing systems, images of known P450 3D structures, table of age-dependent changes in liver microsomal P450 and a tree of representative P450 sequences.
  http://www.icgeb.trieste.it/~p450srv/
- Human Cytochrome P450 Allele Nomenclature Committee.
  http://www.imm.ki.se/CYPalleles/
- Human P450 Metabolism Data Base. A very user-friendly site that gives a wealth of information on P450 multiple forms, drug substrates and inducers/inhibitors of CYPs (all categories with representative literature reference).
  http://www.gentest.com/human_p450_database/index.html
- Cytochrome P450 Clans: a nomenclature for the combination of P450 families into related clusters (clans).
  http://drnelson.utmem.edu/Clans.html

3 INDUCTION AND INHIBITION OF DRUG METABOLISM

LEARNING OBJECTIVES

At the end of this chapter, you should be able to:
- Appreciate the potential of drugs and chemicals to induce and inhibit the enzymes of drug metabolism
- Describe the major role of the cytochromes P450 in induction and inhibition
- Describe the molecular mechanisms of induction of the major cytochromes P450 and the importance of cellular receptors
- Appreciate that inhibition of drug-metabolising enzymes can arise through a variety of different mechanisms
- Assess how induction and inhibition contribute to drug tolerance, variability in drug responses, drug–drug interactions and drug toxicity

3.1 INTRODUCTION

The study of drug metabolism in experimental animals in general and man in particular is ideally studied under strictly controlled conditions, such that we only observe the influence of the normal physiological and biochemical processes that contribute to the metabolism of the drug in question. However, this ideal situation is rarely achieved and the metabolism of drugs is substantially influenced by the deliberate or passive intake of many chemical substances that man is increasingly being exposed to either in his environment, for medical reasons or as a result of his lifestyle. These chemical substances are derived from a variety of sources and include pharmaceutical products, cosmetics, food additives and industrial chemicals. As summarised in Table 3.1, the magnitude of the various chemicals in use today, and hence the potential exposure to man, is staggering.

While it is clear that the ingestion of drugs, and to a certain extent food additives, is a predetermined, conscious act, many of the chemicals in Table 3.1 enter the body by more subtle means, as exemplified by the pollution of food chains by insecticides and the accidental (sometimes intentional) exposure to industrial chemicals and solvents from the environment. The magnitude of this

Classification	Number
Active ingredients of pesticides	1 500
Pharmaceutical products (drugs)	6 000
Food additives with nutritional value	2 500
Food additives to promote product life	3 000
Additional chemicals in use (including industrial chemicals)	50 000

Table 3.1 Estimated chemicals in use today

latter problem is clearly seen in a recent study in the United States, where the Environmental Protection Agency reported that 288 different classes of chemical compounds were identified in domestic drinking water supplies. The food supply also represents an abundant source of chemical additives such as anti-oxidants, colourants, flavour enhancers and stabilisers that the human population is continually exposed to on a daily basis. For example, a recent UK government survey analysed approximately 5000 food products which contained 7000 chemical additives. Put another way, the average dietary intake of food additives in the UK is approximately 8 g/person/day or 2.9 kg/person/year.

From the above considerations, it is clear that man is either intentionally or accidentally exposed to many chemical substances that have the potential to alter drug metabolism. Accordingly, it is the purpose of this chapter to outline the induction and inhibition of drug metabolism by these chemicals and to rationalise, wherever possible, their mode(s) of action on a molecular basis. Other factors affecting drug metabolism (including species, genetic, sex, age and dietary factors) are considered in the following two chapters and the pharmacological, toxicological and clinical implications of altered drug metabolism are considered in subsequent chapters.

3.2 INDUCTION OF DRUG METABOLISM

3.2.1 Induction of drug metabolism in experimental animals

The duration and intensity of pharmacological action of many drugs is primarily dictated by their rate of metabolism and, as a corollary, chemical inducers that modify drug metabolism would be expected to alter the pharmacological effects of drugs. A good example of this phenomenon is the influence of phenobarbitone and benzo[a]pyrene on the metabolism and duration of action of the muscle relaxant, zoxazolamine. As shown in Figure 3.1, zoxazolamine undergoes metabolic hydroxylation at the 6-position by liver homogenates to form a pharmacologically inactive metabolite and, as shown in Table 3.2, pretreatment of experimental animals with either phenobarbitone or the polycyclic aromatic hydrocarbon, benzo[a]pyrene, results in a substantial increase in zoxazolamine metabolism and, consequently, a significant decrease in the paralysis time by the drug.

Clearly, the range of drugs and chemicals that have the ability to induce similar hepatic drug metabolism has been more thoroughly investigated in laboratory animals than in man and, as documented in Table 3.3, many structurally diverse drugs and chemicals have been shown to induce liver drug metabolism in various species.

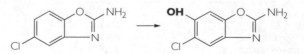

Figure 3.1 Metabolism of zoxazolamine by rat liver homogenates.

Table 3.2 Influence of phenobarbitone or benzo[a]pyrene pretreatment on the metabolism and pharmacological action of zoxazolamine in the rat

Parameter	Control (saline treated)	Phenobarbitone treated[a]	Benzo[a]pyrene treated[b]
Paralysis time (min)	137	62	20
Whole body decay ($t_{1/2}$, min)	102	38	12
Zoxazolamine metabolism (nmol/mg protein/h)	3	14	15

[a] Animals were treated with phenobarbitone (30 mg/kg, i.p.) twice daily for 4 days and killed 24 h after the last injection.
[b] Animals were treated with a single i.p. injection of benzo[a]pyrene (20 mg/kg) 24 h prior to sacrifice.
Adaped from Trevor, A. (1972) In: *Fundamentals of Drug Metabolism and Drug Disposition* (B.N. La Du et al., eds.). Williams and Wilkins, Baltimore.

Table 3.3 Inducers of hepatic drug metabolism in experimental animals

Classification	Example	Use or occurrence
Drugs	Phenobarbitone and most barbiturates	Sedative/hypnotic
	Phenytoin	Anti-convulsant
	Pregnenolone-16α-carbonitrile	Catatoxic steroid
	Rifampicin	Antibiotic
	Triacetyloleandomycin	Antibiotic
	Clofibrate	Hypolipidaemic
Alcohols	Ethanol	Beverage, skin disinfectant
Flavones	5,6-Benzoflavone	Synthetics, citrus fruits
Food additives and nutrients	Butylated hydroxyanisole (BHA), butylated hydroxytoluene (BHT), ethoxyquin	Food antioxidants
	Isosafrole	Oils of sassafras, nutmeg and cinnamon
Halogenated hydrocarbons	2,3,7,8-Tetrachlorodibenzo-p-dioxin (TCDD)	Contaminant of herbicides and defoliants (2,4,5-T)
	3,3',4,4'-Tetrachlorobiphenyl	Insulator in capacitors/transformers
	3,3',4,4',5,5'-Hexabromobiphenyl	Flame retardant
Insecticides	DDT (dichlorodiphenyl trichloroethane)	Agricultural pesticide
	Chlordecone (Kepone)	Organochlorine pesticide
	Piperonyl butoxide	Insecticide synergist
Polycyclic aromatic hydrocarbons	Including 3-methylcholanthrene, phenanthrene, chrysene, 1-2,benzanthracene and benzo[a]pyrene	Environmental pollutants found in industrial and domestic combustion products, cigarette smoke and oil contaminants
Solvents	Toluene and xylenes	Solvents, cleaning agents and degreasers

There is apparently no structure–activity relationship in the ability of these various inducers to stimulate drug metabolism and the only common physico-chemical property is that the majority of these compounds are relatively lipophilic in nature.

3.2.2 Induction of drug metabolism in man

Many currently used drugs of diverse pharmacology and chemical structure are well known to induce either their own metabolism or the biotransformation of other drugs in man (Table 3.4). The list of drugs shown in Table 3.4 is by no means complete and only reflects those drugs for which there is a reasonably strong body of evidence for their ability to induce drug metabolism in man, and almost certainly this list is much longer in reality.

As indicated in Chapter 1, the liver is the major organ responsible for drug metabolism in most species, and as far as man is concerned, a major problem is how to assess the extent of induction of hepatic drug metabolism. Several methods have been proposed to study induction in man and these include increased drug clearance, decreased drug plasma half-life, increased plasma gamma-glutamyl transferase, increased urinary excretion of D-glucaric acid, increased urinary 6β-hydroxycortisol and plasma bilirubin levels. Although none of these methods can unequivocally substantiate the induction of drug metabolism in man, taken collectively, they provide a reasonable indication of induction. Although the mechanism(s) involved in the induction of drug metabolism in man are still being clarified, the induction of specific liver enzymes (particularly the mixed-function

Table 3.4 Therapeutic drugs that induce their own metabolism or the biotransformation of other drugs in man

Classification	Examples
Analeptics	Nikethamide
Analgesic, antipyretic and anti-inflammatory drugs	Antipyrine Phenylbutazone
Antibiotics	Rifampicin
Anticonvulsants	Carbamazepine, Phenytoin
Antifungal drugs	Griseofulvin
Antilipidaemics	Halofenate
Antimalarials	Quinine
Diuretics	Spironolactone
Psychotropic drugs	Chlorimipramine
Sedatives and hypnotics	Amylobarbitone, barbitone, chloral hydrate, cyclobarbitone, dichloralphenazone, glutethimide, hexobarbitone, mandrax (a mixture of methaqualone and diphenyhydramine), meprobamate, phenobarbitone
Steroids	Testosterone
Vitamins	Vitamin C

Adapted from Bowman, W. and Rand, J., *Textbook of Pharmacology* 2nd edn. Blackwell, London (1980).

oxidase enzymes of the endoplasmic reticulum) plays a substantial role and has profound implications in clinical pharmacology and toxicology, as discussed in Chapters 6 and 7.

Clearly then, there are many problems associated with both the assessment and understanding of the basic mechanisms involved in the induction of drug metabolism in man, not the least of which are the ethical considerations. As a consequence of these limitations, much attention has focused on the use of experimental animals in drug induction studies. Although animal studies have proved extremely useful in characterising the phenomena of drug metabolism and its induction, it must always be borne in mind that induction experiments in animals do not always faithfully reproduce all drug effects observed in man.

3.2.3 Role of cytochrome P450 in the induction of drug metabolism

In an attempt to localise the site of induction of drug metabolism, significant advances have been made in considering the role of the liver. As outlined in Chapter 1, the liver serves as the main organ responsible for drug metabolism and it was not entirely unexpected that significant hepatic alterations in the drug metabolising enzyme systems were noted in response to inducing agents. Of particular importance is the hepatic cytochrome P450 enzyme system. Early studies in the mid-1960s clearly showed that both cytochrome P450 and its associated flavoprotein reductase, NADPH-cytochrome P450 reductase, were substantially induced in response to phenobarbitone pretreatment and that this was paralleled by induction of drug metabolism. This observed inductive effect of phenobarbitone was not, however, confined to the enzymes of drug metabolism and other enzymes of the hepatic endoplasmic reticulum were induced, indicative of a general proliferation of this subcellular organelle.

Nevertheless, it soon became clear that induction of drug metabolism was generally accompanied by increases in liver microsomal cytochrome P450 content and, in addition, different inducers did not uniformly increase the metabolism of all drugs to the same extent, i.e. certain inducers did indeed substantially increase drug metabolism, other inducers had little or no effect and, paradoxically, certain 'inducers' actually decreased the metabolism of some drugs investigated. In addition to exhibiting a certain degree of substrate specificity, inducers are well documented to exhibit both stereo- and regioselectivity towards the metabolism of several drugs. This is exemplified by the influence of inducers on the metabolism of the R- and S-isomers of warfarin, both isomers of warfarin being hydroxylated at various positions in the molecule by the cytochrome P450-dependent mixed-function oxidase system of the liver endoplasmic reticulum (Table 3.5).

In view of the extremely broad substrate specificity of liver microsomal cytochrome P450 towards the metabolism of drugs, and the diversity of responses to inducers as outlined above, it was initially proposed that these observations could be rationalised by assuming the existence of more than one form of cytochrome P450. Thus different inducers would have the potential to elevate the levels of a specific sub-population of cytochromes P450, each with a characteristic substrate specificity towards the metabolism of drugs. This concept of cytochrome

Table 3.5 Influence of cytochrome P450 induction on the *in vitro* metabolism of R- and S-warfarin

| | Hydroxylated warfarin metabolites[a] | | | |
| | R-isomer | | S-isomer | |
Inducer	7-OH	8-OH	7-OH	8-OH
Uninduced	0.22	0.04	0.04	0.01
Phenobarbitone	0.36	0.07	0.09	0.02
3-Methylcholanthrene	0.08	0.50	0.05	0.04

[a] Metabolism is expressed as nmol warfarin metabolite formed/nmol cytochrome P450/min

P450 multiplicity has been firmly established in recent years and has had a profound influence on drug metabolism studies. Validation of this latter hypothesis has been achieved largely by the development of techniques enabling the cytochromes P450 to be solubilised and purified from liver endoplasmic reticulum fragments such that structural and functional comparisons of highly purified cytochrome P450 preparations can be assessed and compared. More recently, this latter approach has been replaced by molecular cloning of the relevant cytochrome P450 genes, their expression in cell systems and subsequent substrate specificity characterisation, the majority of which are commercially available.

There are strain differences and tissue differences in expression of these multiple forms, in addition to the presence of more than one form in a given tissue of a given species. The precise reasons why a particular tissue in a particular species expresses a specific and limited complement of cytochromes P450 still awaits resolution, but it is becoming increasingly recognised that tissue-specific transcription factors (including cellular receptors) are likely to play an important role. There is now unambiguous evidence that man, like experimental animals, expresses several cytochrome P450 forms and, furthermore, that many of these enzymes are inducible by drugs and xenobiotics.

3.2.4 Molecular mechanisms of induction of multiple forms of cytochrome P450

In recent years, much effort has been expended in trying to understand the mechanisms underpinning induction of the drug-metabolising enzymes in hepatic tissue. Figure 3.2 shows the functional components of the hepatic mixed-function oxidase system responsible for cytochrome P450-dependent drug metabolism. Accordingly, induction of drug metabolism may arise as a consequence of increased synthesis, decreased degradation, activation of pre-existing components or a combination of these three processes (Table 3.6), although it should be emphasised that the majority of cytochromes P450 are induced at the level of transcriptional activation.

CYP1A1

Much interest has centred on CYP1A1 because of its ability to activate environmental compounds such as the polycyclic aromatic hydrocarbons (PAH) to biologically reactive metabolites that interact with DNA, resulting in chemical

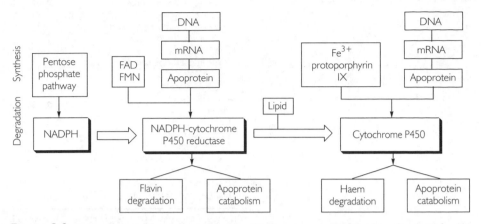

Figure 3.2 Synthesis and degradation of the functional components of the hepatic mixed-function oxidase system.

Table 3.6 Differences in induction mechanisms for cytochromes P450[a]

P450 form	Representative inducer	Main induction mechanism
1A1	Dioxin	Transcription activation by ligand activated Ah receptor
1A2	3-Methylcholanthrene	mRNA stabilisation
2B1/2B2	Phenobarbital	Transcriptional gene activation
2E1	Ethanol, acetone, isoniazid	Protein stabilisation (in part)
3A1	Dexamethasone	Transcriptional gene activation
4A6	Clofibrate	Transcriptional activation, mediated by peroxisome proliferator activated receptor

[a] Modified from Waxman, D.J. and Azaroff, L. (1992) *Biochem. J.* **228**, 577–592.

carcinogenesis. Accordingly, an understanding of CYP1A1 regulation is an important factor in determining and assessing susceptibility to chemical carcinogenesis. CYP1A1 is induced by a large group of environmental chemicals including the polycyclic aromatic hydrocarbons such as 3-methylcholanthrene, β-naphthoflavone, benzo[*a*]pyrene, 2,3,7,8-tetrachlorodibenzo-*p*-dioxin (TCDD, dioxin) amongst others (Table 3.7) and is associated with a specific cytosolic receptor, termed the Ah receptor (AhR). As shown in Figure 3.3, polycyclic aromatic hydrocarbon inducers enter the cell and combine with cytosolic AhR. Inducer-free AhR exists in combination with at least two other proteins (heat shock protein 90 [Hsp90] and AhR interacting protein [AIP]), the function of which is not entirely clear but they are thought to maintain the AhR in a receptive configuration for inducer binding. The inducer–receptor complex translocates to the nucleus where it heterodimerises with the AhR nuclear translocator protein, termed Arnt. This inducer–AhR–Arnt complex (probably in conjunction with other transcription factors) targets a number of genes in the nucleus (including CYP1A1). The interaction

Table 3.7 Polycyclic aromatic hydrocarbon-like inducers of cytochrome P450

Polycyclic aromatic hydrocarbons
   3-methylcholanthrene
   benzo(*a*)pyrene
   benz(*a*)anthracene
   dibenz(*a,h*)anthracene
Phenothiazines
β-Naphthoflavone and other flavones
Plant indoles
   indole-3-acetonitrile
   indole-3-carbinol
Ellipticine
Charcoal-broiled beef
Cigarette smoke
Crude petroleum
Polychlorinated biphenyls
Polybrominated biphenyls
Halogenated dibenzo-*p*-dioxins
Halogenated dibenzofurans

Derived from Okey, A.B. (1990) *Pharmacol. Therapeut.* **45**, 241–298.

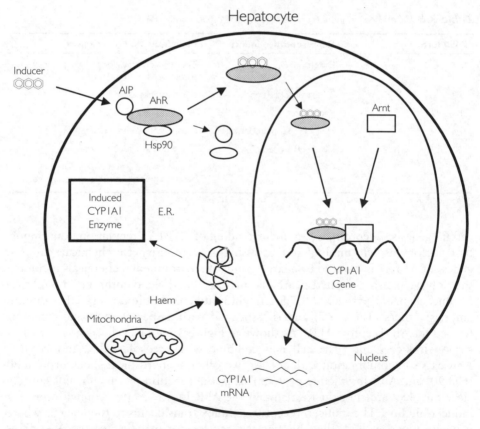

Figure 3.3 Receptor-mediated induction of CYP1A1 by polycyclic aromatic hydrocarbons. Abbreviations used: AIP, Ahr-interacting protein; AhR, aryl hydrocarbon receptor; Hsp90, heat shock protein 90; Arnt, AhR nuclear translocator; E.R., endoplasmic reticulum.

of this inducer complex with the regulatory elements (enhancer/promoter region) of cytochrome P450 responsive genes (primarily CYP1A1) is now reasonably well understood at the molecular level and is a complex interactive system of multiple copies of positive control elements (drug responsive elements, DREs or sometimes called xenobiotic responsive elements, XREs, of the sequence 5'-TNGCGTG which function as transcriptional enhancers, and negative control elements, situated at approximately −1 kilobase upstream of the transcriptional start site in the 5' flanking region of the gene. An initiation complex thereby forms at the CYP1A1 promoter and increases the rate of CYP1A1 mRNA synthesis. Large amounts of newly translated, specific cytochrome P450 protein are then incorporated into the membrane of the hepatic endoplasmic reticulum (along with haem insertion), resulting in the observed induction of metabolism of certain drugs and xenobiotics. It should be noted that CYP1A1 is predominantly expressed in extra-hepatic tissue (particularly human lung) and is present in low amounts in non-induced liver (approximately 2–5% of the total cytochrome P450 content) but increases approximately 8–16-fold on induction, dependent on the species and tissue in question. CYP1A2 is constitutively expressed in human liver in low amounts.

The AhR is a cytosolic protein of molecular weight approximately 88 kda and is a member of a larger family of basic helix–loop–helix/Per–Arnt–Sim (bHLH/PAS) transcription factors. The receptor consists of several functional domains including those for ligand binding, DNA binding, dimerisation, transactivation, nuclear import/export and Hsp90 interaction. It should be recognised that the AhR/Arnt system is not solely dedicated to transcriptional activation of the CYP1A1 gene and many other genes are also activated, including some other xenobiotic metabolising enzymes. The above induction process emphasises a key role for AhR in the induction process, underscored by the observation that certain mouse strains lack this receptor and are comparatively non-responsive to CYP1A1 inducers. Furthermore, AhR gene knockout mice also are non-responsive. Interestingly, studies in AhR null mice have suggested that the receptor regulates normal physiological and developmental pathways, the precise nature and extent of which remains to be fully understood.

The Arnt is a nuclear protein of molecular weight approximately 86 000 kda and, again, consists of distinct functional domains including those for DNA binding, dimerisation, transactivation and nuclear localisation. Arnt null (knockout) mice do not develop past embryonic day 10.5, indicating an important role for this nuclear transcription factor in key developmental processes.

Extensive studies have been carried out on the ability of various polycyclic aromatic hydrocarbons to interact with the above cytosolic receptor and hence induce specific cytochrome P450 variants. For example, Table 3.8 shows the rank order potency of various compounds to inhibit the binding of 3-methylcholanthrene to the cytosolic receptor. From this table it is seen that 2,3,7,8-tetrachlorodibenzo-p-dioxin (TCDD or dioxin) is a potent inhibitor of 3-methylcholanthrene binding to the cytosolic receptor (i.e. has a high affinity) and, in general, the data in Table 3.8 correlate well with the relative potency of these compounds to induce

Table 3.8 Potency of various compounds as competitors of binding of 3-methylcholanthrene to the mouse hepatic cytosolic receptor

Competitor	Competitor concentration giving 50% inhibition of 3-methylcholanthrene binding (M)[a]
2,3,7,8-Tetrachlorodibenzo-p-dioxin	0.3×10^{-9}
Dibenz[a,h]anthracene	0.1×10^{-8}
Dibenz[a,c]anthracene	0.3×10^{-8}
β-Naphthoflavone	0.1×10^{-7}
Benzo[a]pyrene	0.1×10^{-7}
Benz[a]anthracene	0.5×10^{-7}
6-Aminochrysene	0.8×10^{-7}
Pregnenolone-16α-carbonitrile	0.1×10^{-6}
Anthracene	0.8×10^{-6}

[a] 3-Methylcholanthrene concentration was 10 nM.
Adapted from Okey, A.B. and Vella, L.M. (1982) *Eur. J. Biochem.* **127**, 39–47.

CYP1A1. In addition, it should be noted that certain strains of mice are non-responsive to these inducers and are characterised by an absence of the cytosolic receptor.

CYP2Bs

Treatment of experimental animals with phenobarbitone (and related agents, Table 3.9) results in a substantial increase in the hepatic levels of translatable polysomal mRNA for some cytochromes P450, particularly CYP2B1. Specific complementary DNA probes (cDNA) to cytochrome P450 mRNA have been synthesised and, using cDNA–mRNA hybridisation techniques, it has been shown conclusively that a few hours after phenobarbitone pretreatment, a substantial increase in the level of mRNA coding for cytochrome P4502B1 is observed. This mRNA induction is accompanied by increases in intranuclear RNAs that represent precursors to cytochrome P450 and mRNA.

An interesting example of phenobarbitone-dependent gene regulation is in the differential regulation of CYPs 2B1 and 2B2. These two closely related isoenzymes share an overall 97% amino acid sequence similarity with only 14 residues different out of a total of 491. One of these variable regions is in exon 7 in residues 344–349 as

CYP2B2–Ser–His–Arg–Leu–Pro–Thr–

CYP2B1–Ser–His–Arg–Pro–Pro–Ser–

Table 3.9 Drugs and chemicals that act as phenobarbitone-type inducers of cytochromes P450

Phenobarbitone and several barbiturates
Phenytoin
DDT
Pentamethylbenzene
Polychlorinated biphenyls (PCBs) with *ortho* chlorines
2-Acetylaminofluorene

Derived from Okey, A.B. (1990) *Pharmacol. Therapeut.* **45**, 241–298.

Knowing these small differences in amino acid sequence, specific oligonucleotide probes can be chemically synthesised for the above two enzymes, thus yielding an analytical method to determine the influence of phenobarbitone on these closely related enzymes. This type of molecular analysis has yielded the information that, even though the sequences of CYP2B1 and CYP2B2 are almost identical, their regulation by phenobarbitone is very different (CYP2B1 is induced, CYP2B2 is not) with the functional importance that CYP2B1 and 2B2 exhibit different rates of substrate biotransformation (CYP2BI is usually more active than CYP2B2) and hence contribute to differential activation/deactivation of xenobiotics, including cyclophosphamide amongst several others. In man, CYP2B6 is the only member of the CYP2B family expressed in liver, whereas CYP2B7 is mainly expressed in human lung.

It would appear that the major inductive effect of phenobarbitone in the liver is to increase specific mRNA levels by increasing gene transcription, rather than stabilising pre-existing levels of protein precursors or increased translational efficiency. Much effort has been expended in recent years in trying to understand the molecular mechanisms whereby phenobarbitone induces cytochromes P450 and it is only very recently that this has begun to clarify, with two distinct mechanisms emerging, one in bacteria and the other in eukaryotic systems. The phenobarbital-inducible CYP102A1 in *Bacillus megaterium* was historically the first to be characterised, with the key feature being a 17 bp sequence in the 5′-flanking region (termed the Barbie Box) which binds a repressor protein termed Bm3R1 (Figure 3.4(a)). In the resting state, this repressor protein suppresses CYP102A1 gene expression, a suppression that is removed by exposure of the bacterium to phenobarbitone. Therefore, to be strictly correct, the mechanism of induction in this case is de-repression.

Although mammalian genes in the CYP2B family do contain homologous sequences to the Barbie Box in *Bacillus megaterium*, it would appear that this region does not confer phenobarbitone responsiveness, as deletion or mutation in the Barbie Box still retain phenobarbitone responsiveness. For the mammalian CYP2B sub-family, the critical regulatory region for induction is a 51 bp sequence situated approximately 2 kbp downstream of the transcription initiation site and termed the phenobarbitone-responsive enhancer module (PBREM, Figure 3.4(b)). The PBREM consists of two nuclear receptor binding sites (NR1 and NR2), which are imperfect direct repeats spaced by 4 bp, otherwise known as a DR4 motif. This PBREM recognises and binds a heterodimer of two nuclear receptors termed the constitutive androstane receptor (CAR) and the retinoid X receptor (RXR). CAR is an unusual receptor in that it is transcriptionally active in the absence of bound ligand, and upon binding of its steroid ligands (androstanol [5α-androstan-3α-ol] and androstenol [5α-androst-16-en-3α-ol]) is transcriptionally inactive. Although the precise molecular mechanisms whereby phenobarbitone interacts with this transcription factor complex still need clarifying, it would appear that the barbiturate (and other related inducers of the CYP2Bs) relieves the transcriptional repression of CAR produced by androstenol and androstanol. Recent studies have demonstrated that this phenobarbitone-dependent, CAR-mediated activation of the PBREM transcription unit operates in human liver CYP2B6.

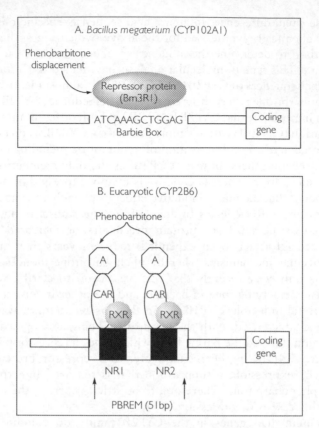

Figure 3.4 Regulation of cytochrome P450 genes by phenobarbitone. (a) *Bacillus megaterium* CYP102A1 and (b) eucaryotic CYP2B genes. Abbreviations used: CAR, constitutive androstane receptor; RXR, retinoid X receptor; NR, nuclear receptor binding site; A, constitutive CAR steroid ligands (androstanol and androstenol).

Although the above discussion substantiates a role for CAR-mediated induction of CYP2B genes by phenobarbitone, it is currently not entirely clear if this represents the sole mechanism. For example, recent studies have highlighted the importance of the glucocorticoid receptor (GR) in regulating CYP2B genes in the mouse, in that GR null (knockout) mice had a substantially lower level of constitutive CYP2B and they were refractory to induction by both dexamethasone and pregnane 16α-carbonitrile, thereby suggesting a role for the GR in the induction process.

CYP2E1

CYP2E1 plays a predominant role in toxicology as many of its substrates are bioactivated to reactive metabolites, including paracetamol and low molecular weight substrates such as nitrosamines, benzene, carbon tetrachloride and ethylene glycol, resulting in liver and kidney toxicity. The administration of ethanol (alcohol) to experimental animals and man results in the induction of the bio-transformation of drugs, xenochemicals and the oxidation of ethanol itself, suggesting that ethanol induces a specific form of cytochrome P450. This turned out to be the case and ethanol (and other compounds such as imidazole, isoniazid, acetone and pyrazole) induces the CYP2E1 enzyme. The amount of CYP2E1 protein is 4-fold higher in the liver derived from alcoholics compared to non-drinkers and the plasma clearance of chlorzoxazone (a CYP2E1 substrate) in man is doubled in individuals imbibing excessive amounts of alcohol (>300 g/day).

Interestingly, the induction of CYP2E1 arises through multiple mechanisms, depending on the induction stimulus and includes transcriptional, translational and post-translational mechanisms. Although our current knowledge on the detailed molecular mechanisms of CYP2E1 gene regulation are not as well developed as the CYP1A1 and CYP2B genes, it appears that the predominant xenobiotic-dependent induction mechanism appears to be via stabilisation and inhibition of degradation of the CYP2EI apoprotein.

CYP3A

Members of the cytochrome P450 3A (CYP3A) sub-family are highly expressed in most experimental animals and human liver/intestine and play a pivotal role in the metabolism of clinically used drugs and certain toxic environmental chemicals. CYP3A4 is predominantly expressed in human liver and intestine where it comprises between 30 and 50% of the total cytochrome P450 population in these tissues. This isoform is highly inducible in man by synthetic glucocorticoids (dexamethasone), macrolide antibiotics (rifampicin) and phenobarbitone, amongst others, and has been estimated to be responsible for approximately 60% of the cytochrome P450-mediated metabolism of pharmaceuticals in therapeutic use today, in addition to metabolising a number of endogenous compounds, such as testosterone, and environmental xenobiotics, such as aflatoxins. Accordingly, it is not surprising that a substantial amount of effort has been expended in attempting to understand the molecular mechanisms of regulation of this important enzyme.

Currently, three human CYP3A enzymes have been identified, namely CYP3A4, CYP3A5 and CYP3A7. The CYP3A sub-family is the major cytochrome P450 expressed in human liver at all stages of development with CYP3A7 predominating in foetal liver and CYP3A4 in adult liver. However, the CYP3As are also expressed in other tissues. CYP3A5 is the major CYP3A in the stomach and both CYP3A4 and CYP3A5 mRNA have been detected by PCR in all regions of the digestive tract. CYP3A4 is the major CYP3A isoform in the liver and the small intestine, whereas CYP3A5 is the main isoform in the human colon. CYP3A4 metabolises aflatoxin B_1 in human small bowel enterocytes, resulting in the formation of intracellular aflatoxin B_1 molecular adducts which pass out in the stool as enterocytes are continuously sloughed off. Otherwise, the reactive metabolite may be absorbed into the systemic circulation and have the potential to form carcinogenic adducts in the liver. Whereas the expression of CYP3A4 in the small intestine is a protective mechanism in the case of aflatoxin B_1, the presence of CYP3A4 in enterocytes suggests that it may be involved in the first-pass metabolism of drugs, thereby limiting the systemic absorption of orally administered drugs. For example, 50% of an oral dose of cyclosporin A undergoes CYP3A4-dependent hydroxylation, thereby contributing to the poor oral bioavailability of the drug in man, a situation that can be exacerbated by the inducibility of the enzyme in the small intestine. CYP3A7 has only been detected in the liver and CYP3A5 appears to be constitutively expressed in the adult kidney.

The CYP3As are responsible for the metabolism of a wide range of drugs and other chemicals in man and is highly inducible by drugs and both synthetic/natural steroids in liver (Table 3.10). Regulation of CYP3A genes is complex, mainly due to the plethora of regulatory elements found in both the distal enhancer and proximal promoter (Figure 3.5 and Table 3.11). In an analogous manner to the CYP1A1 and CYP2B genes, cellular receptors play an important role in regulation of CYP3A gene expression, the most important of which is the pregnane X receptor (PXR). The PXR plays an important role in CYP3A4 gene regulation for several xenobiotic and endogenous steroid inducers in several species, first identified in the mouse and subsequently in rat, rabbit and man. The PXR is a member of the nuclear receptor family, the important structural features being a ligand (inducer)-binding domain and a DNA-binding domain.

In man and other species, a PXR/retinoid X receptor (RXR) heterodimer is essential for the activation of CYP3A4 reporter gene constructs by xenobiotics and naturally occurring pregnane steroids. In addition, two further receptors mediate induction of the CYP3As, namely the glucocorticoid receptor and the constitutive

Table 3.10 Substrates and inducers of human liver CYP3A4

Substrates	Inducers
Aflatoxin B_1	Carbamazepine
Alfentanil	Dexamethasone
Codeine	Fexofenadine
Cyclophosphamide	Hypericum (St John's wort)
Cyclosporin	Lovastatin
Dextromethorphan	Methylprednisolone
Diazepam	Metyrapone
Erythromycin	PCN
Lidocaine	Phenobarbital
Loratidine	Phenytoin
Midazolam	Phenylbutazone
Nifedipine	Prednisone
Omeprazole	Rifampicin
Ritonavir	Sulfinpyrazole
Tamoxifen	Spironolactone
Terfenadine	Troglitazone
Verapamil	Troleandomycin

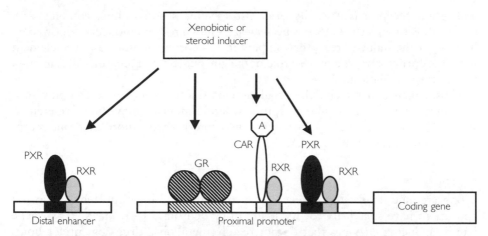

Figure 3.5 Receptor-dependent regulation of the CYP3A4 gene. Abbreviations used: PXR, pregnane X receptor; RXR, retinoid X receptor; GR, glucocorticoid receptor; CAR, constitutive androstane receptor; A, constitutive CAR steroid ligands (androstanol and androstenol). Xenobiotic or steroid inducers can bind either comparatively selectively to one of the receptor systems or promiscuously to more than one receptor with differing affinities. The receptor–inducer complex binds to specific regions in either the distal enhancer or proximal promoter modules, as dictated by the DNA-binding domain of the receptors.

Table 3.11 Regulatory motifs in CYP3A promoters

AP-3	Consensus sequence recognised by the gene activating factor, Activating Protein 3
BTE	Basal Transcription Element involved in maintenance of basal level of transcription in many genes, possibly through the BTE Binding Protein (BTEB), located in the liver
CAAT Box	Consensus sequence present in many genes and binds the liver specific protein C/EBP (CCAAT enhancer binding protein) and the ubiquitous transcription factor CP1 (CCAAT-protein-1) . . . has a major role in determining the efficiency of the promoter
CACCC box	Located upstream of the CAAT box and is thought to be involved in transcriptional activation. Known to bind Sp-1
ERE/PRE/GRE	Response elements with similar consensus sequences. Binding of the ER, PR and GR receptors involved in both positive and negative regulation of gene transcription in response to estrogens, progestogens and glucocortoids
HNF-4 and HNF-5	Regulatory motifs (hepatocyte-specific, nuclear transcription factors) that bind liver-specific transcription factors HNF-4 and HNF-5. Also involved in the regulation of CYP2B genes (HNF-4) and transferrin gene (HNF-5)
Octamer motif	Conserved motif present in many genes (including CYP1A1), binding members of the Octamer factors family, resulting in the up/down regulation of responsive genes
TATA box	Found in all eukaryotic genes and is essential for transcription. Recognised by the TATA binding protein (TBP)
p53	Consensus sequence that binds the tumour suppressor protein, p53
ER_6 motif	Two everted copies of the AG(G/T)TCA motif, separated by 6 nucleotides. Binds the PXR/RXR receptor complex and activates xenobiotic-dependent gene transcription in CYP3A4, CYP3A7 and CYP3A23

androstane receptor (CAR), the latter also forming a heterodimer complex with the RXR. Although the CAR has been clearly shown to bind inducers, followed by binding of the inducer–receptor complex to the corresponding response element in CYP3A promoters, the precise role of the glucocorticoid receptor still remains a matter for speculation.

Thus, taken collectively, the regulation of CYP3A genes is a complex process, involving several cellular receptors, wherein inducers may show preferential specificity for one receptor or promiscuously interact with more than one receptor, as summarised in Figure 3.5.

CYP4A

Clofibrate (and its fibrate congeners) is a clinically used hypolipidaemic drug and appears to have specificity for induction of cytochromes P450 in the CYP4 gene family, inducing enzymes that do not readily metabolise drugs but prefer lipids (particularly fatty acids) as substrates. Recent work has identified, cloned and sequenced a member of the steroid hormone superfamily of receptors, termed the

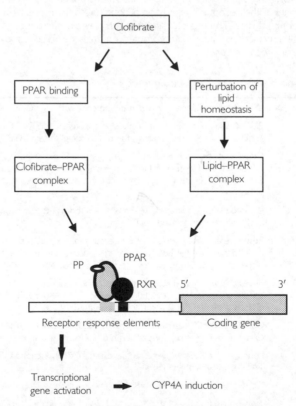

Figure 3.6 Regulation of cytochrome P450 4 family genes by the peroxisome proliferator activated receptor. Abbreviations used: PP, peroxisome proliferator (clofibrate); PPAR, peroxisome proliferator receptor; RXR, retinoid X receptor, the dimerisation partner for PPAR.

peroxisome proliferator activated receptor (PPAR), so called because clofibrate belongs to a large class of compounds known as the peroxisome proliferators. This PPAR consists of two domains, a ligand-binding region that binds clofibrate and a DNA-binding region that binds to the regulatory elements of the responsive genes in the CYP4 family (the interaction with CYP4A6 has been relatively well characterised) as demonstrated in Figure 3.6. It is interesting to note that fatty acids can act as natural ligands for this PPAR and, at present, it is not clear if the CYP4 family induction arises solely from drug–PPAR interaction or clofibrate-dependent perturbation of lipid homeostasis and subsequent lipid activation of the receptor or a combination of these two mechanisms (Figure 3.6).

The above discussion has centred on different types of cytochrome P450 inducers as if every inducer only induces one particular sub-family of enzymes. Whereas this is true for some inducers it most certainly is not true for all of the inducers known to date and it must be borne in mind that certain xenobiotics will induce several sub-families within the same family and even in totally different families.

3.2.5 Induction of extrahepatic drug metabolism

Although the liver is the main organ responsible for drug metabolism in most species, significant activities are present in extrahepatic tissues including lung, kidney, skin, intestinal mucosa, and many other tissues. Whereas the liver appears to be a particularly sensitive target organ for the induction of the drug metabolising enzymes in general, and cytochrome P450 in particular, the inductive response in extrahepatic tissues is more variable. Extrahepatic enzyme induction depends not only on the nature of the inducing agent and the extrahepatic tissue but also on the particular drug substrate under investigation. For example, Table 3.12 shows that cigarette smoke (containing polycyclic aromatic hydrocarbon inducing agents) substantially increases the hydroxylation of benzo[a]pyrene in lung and placenta and is a less effective inducing agent in the intestine. Similarly, induction of phenacetin metabolism in the lung was only 5% of that observed with benzo[a]pyrene metabolism in the same tissue.

Although many extrahepatic cytochromes P450 are induced by drugs and chemicals, it is absolutely clear that many extrahepatic cytochromes P450 are regulated by endogenous compounds and hormones (Table 3.13). Practically all of these cytochromes P450 are involved with the biotransformation of physiologically important compounds and the regulatory mechanisms seem to involve ACTH-dependent increased levels of cAMP in many instances and a cAMP-dependent

Table 3.12 Induction of phenacetin and benzo[a]pyrene metabolism by cigarette smoke in extrahepatic tissues of the rat

Enzyme activity	Induction (% of control value)			
	Liver	Intestine	Lung	Placenta
Phenacetin de-ethylation	20	100	60	–
Benzo[a]pyrene hydroxylation	120	120	1200	500

Table 3.13 Constitutive cytochromes P450 regulated by endogenous compounds[a]

Tissue	Cytochrome P450 species induced	Endogenous inducer/regulator[b]
Adrenal	CYP11A1, CYP11B1, CYP17, CYP21A1	ACTH
Ovary	CYP11A1	FSH
Ovary	CYP17	LH
Ovary	CYP19	FSH
Testis	CYP11A1	LH
Leydig cell	CYP17	LH
Kidney	25OHVITD$_3$1α	PTH

[a] Derived from Okey, A.B. (1990) *Pharmacol. Therapeut.* **45**, 241–298.
[b] Abbreviations used: ACTH, adrenocorticotrophic hormone; FSH, follicle stimulating hormone; LH, lutenising hormone; PTH, parathyroid hormone; 25OHVITD$_3$1α, 25-hydroxy-vitamin D$_3$-1α-hydroxylase.

transcriptional activation of the cognate genes. At present, it is not clear if cAMP directly activates cytochrome P450 gene transcription or if cAMP-regulatable proteins are necessary for induction. These SHIP (steroid hydroxylase inducing proteins) mediators have remained elusive to isolate and characterise but remain a conceptually attractive hypothesis involving trans-activation of an enhancer element in the regulatory (5-flanking) region of the corresponding cytochrome P450 genes. In general terms, the cytochromes P450 discussed above are usually not induced by xenobiotics and this is a very useful separation as these endogenous cytochromes P450 are essential to survival and reproduction of the organism.

3.2.6 Induction of non-cytochrome P450 drug-metabolising enzymes

Although cytochrome P450 is an important enzymatic determinant of drug metabolism, it is by no means the only drug metabolising enzyme whose levels are induced in response to a chemical or drug challenge. Indeed, most of the enzymes

Table 3.14 Induction of drug-metabolising enzymes

Enzyme	Inducer
Epoxide hydrolase	2-Acetylaminofluorene, aldrin, Arochlor 1254, dieldrin, ethoxyquin, isosafrole, 3-methylcholanthrene, phenobarbitone, *trans*-stilbene oxide
Glucuronosyl transferase	Dieldrin, isosafrole, 3-methylcholanthrene, phenobarbitone, polychlorinated biphenyls, 2,3,7,8-tetrachlorodibenzo-*p*-dioxin
NADPH-cytochrome P450 reductase	2-Acetylaminofluorene, dieldrin, isosafrole, phenobarbitone, polychlorinated biphenyls, *trans*-stilbene oxide
Glutathione-*S*-transferase	2-Acetylaminofluorene, 3-methylcholanthrene, phenobarbitone, 2,3,7,8-tetrachlorodibenzo-*p*-dioxin, *trans*-stilbene oxide
Cytochrome b$_5$	2-Acetylaminofluorene, butylated hydroxytoluene, griseofulvin

involved in drug metabolism are induced to various extents by a structurally diverse group of chemicals and drugs and some examples of this are shown in Table 3.14.

In general, the above inducers are relatively non-specific in that they cause a general proliferation of the hepatic endoplasmic reticulum membrane or of the enzymes of drug metabolism. However, it should be pointed out that some of the enzymes shown in Table 3.14 exist in multiple forms (e.g. the glucuronosyl transferases) or as homo/heterodimers of two sub-units (e.g. the glutathione-S-transferases). Accordingly, the induction of UDP-glucuronosyl transferase is highly dependent on the nature of the inducer under consideration. Induction of this latter enzyme with phenobarbitone results in the induction of a form of the transferase that preferentially utilises chloroamphenicol as substrate whereas induction with 3-methylcholanthrene results in a transferase that has a specificity for 3-hydroxy-benzo[a]pyrene as substrate. In a similar manner, there is evidence to suggest that the different sub-units of glutathione-S-transferase are differentially induced by phenobarbitone. Therefore, the induction of non-cytochrome P450 enzymes responsible for drug metabolism (particularly the UDP-glucuronosyl transferases and the glutathione-S-transferases) impose another level of control on the overall metabolic fate of a drug.

3.3 INHIBITION OF DRUG METABOLISM

A major concern of clinical pharmacologists is the area of drug–drug interactions in which two or more drugs are co-administered, resulting in either therapeutic incompatibility or toxic reactions. Although the 'blunderbuss' approach to polypharmacy has significantly diminished in recent years, many patients are still treated simultaneously with a combination of different drugs. For example a recent study of 138 randomly selected i.v. solutions has shown that 24% of these solutions contained two drugs and 14% contained five or more drugs. Just as one drug can induce the metabolism of a second drug, as discussed in the previous section, the inhibition of drug metabolism by other drugs or xenobiotics is a well-recognised phenomenon. Accordingly, it is the purpose of this section to focus on well-defined examples of the inhibition of drug metabolism, particularly at the level of liver cytochrome P450. This inhibition of drug metabolism by drugs or xenobiotics can take place in several ways, including the destruction of pre-existing enzymes, inhibition of enzyme synthesis or by complexing and thus inactivating the drug metabolising enzyme. The reader is also referred to Chapters 4 and 5 where additional consideration is given to inhibition of drug metabolism and to Chapters 6 and 7 where the pharmacological, toxicological and clinical implications of this phenomenon are discussed in detail.

3.3.1 Inhibition of drug metabolism by competitive/non-competitive co-substrates

The drug-metabolising enzymes may be viewed as being promiscuous, in that their substrate specificity is rarely absolute for one particular drug, but rather exhibit

Table 3.15 Inhibitors of human CYP3A4

Inhibitor	K_I (μM)	Type of inhibition
Clotrimazole	0.00025–0.15	Competitive
Ketoconazole	0.015–8.0	Non-competitive, mixed
Ritonavir	0.017	Mixed
Saquinavir	0.7	Competitive
Nicardipine	8.0	Competitive

Derived from Thummel, K. and Wilkinson, G. (1998), *Ann. Rev. Pharmacol. Toxicol.*, **38**, 389–430.

relatively broad substrate specificities. The outcome of this in clinical practice is that two (or more) drugs can compete for the same drug metabolising enzyme and, dependent on their relative affinities and inhibitory potencies, can result in inhibition of one of the drugs. This phenomenon has been extensively studied for CYP3A4, the major human liver cytochrome P450 responsible for the oxidation of the majority of drugs used in the clinic today. Of crucial importance here is the inhibitory potency of such drugs and, as shown in Table 3.15, some drugs are of sufficiently high potency that peak plasma levels in normal clinical usage encompass the inhibitory concentration range. Normally, a K_I value in the low μM range would be anticipated to be inhibitors, whereas it is uncommon for inhibition to result for drugs which have K_I values greater than approximately $50\,\mu M$.

3.3.2 Inhibition of drug metabolism by destruction of hepatic cytochrome P450

Many therapeutic drugs and environmental xenobiotics have the ability to destroy cytochrome P450 in the liver by a variety of mechanisms. For example it has been known for several years that xenobiotics containing an olefinic (C=C) or acetylenic (C≡C) function are porphyrinogenic, resulting in the formation of green pigments in the liver. Some representative examples are given in Table 3.16. The chemical nature of these green pigments has recently been identified in most instances as alkylated or substrate–haem adducts derived from cytochrome P450. Interestingly, the majority of these olefinic and acetylenic compounds are relatively inert *per se* and require metabolic activation by cytochrome P450 itself

Table 3.16 Inhibitors of the drug-metabolising enzymes: drugs and xenobiotics that destroy hepatic cytochrome P450

Olefinic derivatives	Acetylenic derivatives
Allobarbital	Acetylene
Allylisopropylacetamide	Ethchlorvynol
Aprobarbital	Ethynylestradiol
Ethylene	Norethindrone
Fluoroxene	
Secobarbital	
Vinyl chloride	

(prior to adduct formation), and are therefore classified as 'suicide substrates' of the haemoprotein. It should be pointed out that the above suicide substrates are relatively selective towards cytochrome P450 in that cytochrome b_5 concentrations (the other haemoprotein of the hepatic endoplasmic reticulum membrane) are usually not affected by these porphyrinogenic xenobiotics.

A major consequence of haem modification by the above compounds is a significant and sustained drop in the levels of functional cytochrome P450, which in turn results in a reduction in the capacity of the liver to metabolise drugs. In addition, it would appear likely that different hepatic cytochromes P450 exhibit differential susceptibilities to destruction by olefinic xenobiotics. The primary target of olefinic drug-induced loss of functional activity is at the haem locus and is substantiated by the observation that the administration of exogenous haem substantially restored both the hepatic cytochrome P450 content and drug metabolising activity after allylisopropylacetamide treatment, a compound well known to destroy cytochrome P450.

The above suicidal activation of olefinic and acetylenic drugs to active metabolites resulting in cytochrome P450 haem destruction has profound pharmacological implications. For example, pretreatment of experimental animals with allylisopropylacetamide results in a significant increase in both hexobarbitone-induced sleeping time and zoxazolamine-induced paralysis time (Table 3.17), both these drugs undergoing cytochrome P450-dependent metabolism.

These results also support the concept that allylisopropylacetamide preferentially destroys a phenobarbitone-inducible cytochrome P450 enzyme in that hexobarbitone (a preferred substrate of this enzyme) sleeping time was increased six-fold, whereas zoxazolamine (not readily metabolised by this cytochrome P450 variant) paralysis time was only increased two-fold.

Accordingly, inhibition of drug metabolism by olefinic and acetylenic drugs and xenobiotics depends not only on the chemical nature of the drug itself but also on the prevailing complement of cytochrome P450 enzymes and their substrate specificities. It should be pointed out that, although the above examples have highlighted the ability of allylisopropylacetamide to destroy cytochrome P450 and consequently inhibit drug metabolism, many drugs have similar properties. In view of the common occurrence of olefinic and acetylenic groups in pharmaceutical products in use today, it is clear that many drug–drug interactions may be rationalised at the level of cytochrome P450 destruction.

Table 3.17 Influence of allylisopropylacetamide (AIA) on the pharmacological activity of hexobarbitone and zoxazolamine

	Control	AIA pretreated
Hexobarbitone sleeping time (min)	37.8 ± 2.0	235.6 ± 27.8
Zoxazolamine paralysis time (min)	257.6 ± 10.5	477.8 ± 31.5

Rats were given either hexobarbitone (150 mg/kg, i.p.) or zoxazolamine (100 mg/kg, i.p.) 11 h after allylisopropylacetamide (300 mg/kg, s.c.).
Adapted from Unseld, F. and DeMatteis, F. (1978) *Int. J. Biochem.* **9**, 865–869.

3.3.3 Metal ions and hepatic cytochrome P450

Related to the above inhibitory effects of olefinic and acetylenic compounds on drug metabolism is the ability of metal ions to substantially inhibit functional oxidase activity. The influence of metal ions on drug metabolism activities is considered in Chapter 5 and it is informative to concentrate on the role of cobalt in drug biotransformation reactions. As shown in Table 3.18, cobalt (in the form of cobalt–haem) has a pronounced influence on both drug metabolism and the biosynthesis/degradation of hepatic haem. In particular, subsequent to cobalt pretreatment, drug metabolism was substantially decreased, as was the hepatic microsomal content of cytochrome P450 and total haem. These results can be rationalised by the observation that cobalt has a pronounced inhibitory effect on the rate-limiting step of haem biosynthesis (δ-aminolevulinic acid synthetase) and additionally causes a substantial increase in haem catabolism, as reflected in the six-fold increase in haem oxygenase activity. The importance of these latter two enzymes in the synthesis and degradation of cytochrome P450–haem is shown in Figure 3.7.

Therefore, in contrast to the olefinic and acetylenic drugs described above that act primarily by modifying existing cytochrome P450–haem, metal ions such as cobalt exert their inhibitory influences on drug metabolism by modulating both the synthesis and degradation of the haem prosthetic group of cytochrome P450.

3.3.4 Inhibition of drug metabolism by compounds forming inactive complexes with hepatic cytochrome P450

In addition to modulating the synthesis/degradation of hepatic cytochrome P450, certain classes of drugs and xenobiotics can inhibit drug metabolism by totally

Table 3.18   Acute effects of cobalt–haem on hepatic drug metabolism and haem biosynthesis

Activity	Saline control	Cobalt–haem treated
Ethylmorphine demethylase (pmol HCHO/mg/h)	0.56 ± 0.06	0.06 ± 0.02
Aniline hydroxylase (nmol 4-aminophenol/mg/h)	89.4 ± 6.9	32.8 ± 3.0
Microsomal haem (nmol/mg)	1.85 ± 0.04	0.89 ± 0.05
Cytochrome P450 (nmol/mg)	0.80 ± 0.04	0.19 ± 0.03
Cytochrome b_5 (nmol/mg)	0.35 ± 0.01	0.23 ± 0.01
Haem oxygenase (nmol bilirubin/mg/h)	2.65 ± 0.11	15.62 ± 0.09
δ-Aminolevulinate synthetase (nmol product/mg/h)	0.20 ± 0.05	0.02 ± 0.01

A single dose of cobalt–haem (125 pmol/kg, s.c.) was given to rats and the above data determined 72 h later. Adapted from Drummond, G. and Kappas, H. (1982) *Proc. Nat. Acad. Sci. (USA)* **79**, 2384–2388.

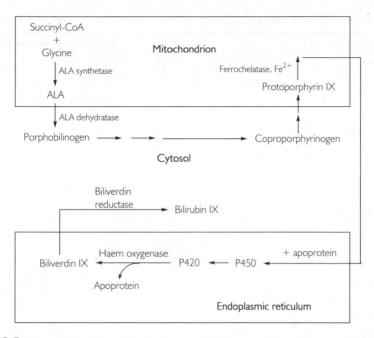

Figure 3.7 Biosynthesis of hepatic cytochrome P450 haem. Abbreviation used: ALA, δ-amino-levulinic acid.

different means, e.g. by forming spectrally detectable, inactive complexes with the haemoprotein. These compounds are substrates of cytochrome P450 and require metabolism to exert their full inhibitory effects, in a similar manner to the olefinic and acetylenic drugs described earlier. However, unlike the latter group of drugs, inhibitors forming complexes are metabolised by cytochrome P450, forming a metabolic intermediate (or product) that binds tightly to the haemoprotein that originally formed it, thus preventing its further participation in drug metabolism and forming the basis of the observed inhibition. Examples of this class of inhibitors are shown in Table 3.19.

A direct comparison of the inhibition of drug metabolism by many of the drugs shown in Table 3.19 is complicated by the observation that the parent drugs themselves exhibit some degree of competitive or non-competitive inhibition. However it is clear that pre-incubation of the inhibitor with liver homogenates (i.e. metabolism) results in a substantial increase in the inhibitory action of these drugs. Furthermore, the above observations are reflected *in vivo* where it has been observed that pretreatment of experimental animals with these inhibitors results in a substantial increase in both hexobarbital narcosis and zoxazolamine paralysis times.

Mechanistic studies on the inhibition by the above xenobiotics have mainly been attempted with amphetamine and methylenedioxybenzene compounds. Although the precise nature of the inhibitory, reactive metabolites responsible for the

Table 3.19 Drugs and xenobiotics inhibiting drug metabolism by complexing with cytochrome P450

Nitrogenous compounds	Non-nitrogenous compounds
Amphetamine	Isosafrole
Benactyzine	Piperanol
Cimetidine	Piperonyl butoxide
Dapsone	Safrole
Desimipramine	Sesamol
2-Diethylaminoethyl-2,2-diphenylvalerate (SKF 525 A)	
2,5-Dimethoxy-4-methylamphetamine (STP)	
Diphenhydramine	
Fenfluramine	
Isoniazid	
Methadone	
Methamphetamine	
Nortriptyline	
Oleandomycin	
Phenmetrazine	
Propoxyphene	
Sulfanilamide	
Triacetyloleandomycin	

observed inhibition has not been absolutely delineated, there is strong evidence to support the theory that amphetamines act through the nitro (or nitroxide) metabolite and the methylenedioxybenzene derivatives are activated to a reactive carbene and subsequent ligation to cytochrome P450 (Figure 3.8). The complexes thus formed exhibit distinctive spectral characteristics and normally absorb maximally at 448–456 nm with the reduced (ferrous) form of cytochrome P450.

An interesting example of the above inhibition of drug metabolism is seen with the antibiotic triacetyloleandomycin. Triacetyloleandomycin (similar in structure to erythromycin) is widely used in man to treat patients who are sensitive to penicillin and several reports have appeared where the administration of this antibiotic produces severe drug–drug reactions. For example, concomitant administration of triacetyloleandomycin with oral contraceptives may produce liver cholestasis, ischemic incidents with ergotamine, neurologic signs of carbamazepine intoxication and theophylline intoxication, suggesting that triacetyloleandomycin may somehow decrease the metabolism of these drugs in humans. Triacetyloleandomycin is interesting in that it induces its own demethylation and subsequent oxidation to a metabolite that forms a stable complex which absorbs at 456 nm with ferrous cytochrome P450 in the liver. On prolonged usage, this compound then inhibits drug oxidation and modulates the pharmacological activity of hexobarbitone (Table 3.20).

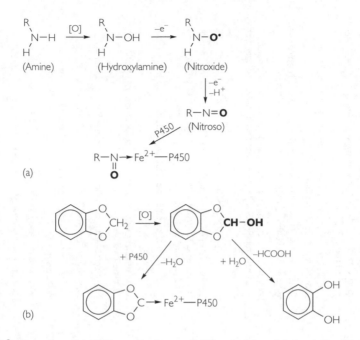

Figure 3.8 Formation of inhibitory cytochrome P450 complexes. (a) Amphetamines, (b) methylenedioxybenzene compounds.

Accordingly, it has been postulated that the drug–drug interactions referred to above can be rationalised by complexation and subsequent inhibition of cytochrome P450. Interestingly, a related antibiotic, oleandomycin (three free hydroxyl groups, not *N*-acetylated), exhibits partially similar properties to triacetyloleandomycin in that oleandomycin can also induce its own cytochrome P450-dependent metabolism. However, compared to triacetyloleandomycin, oleandomycin is both a weaker inducer of microsomal enzymes and also a much poorer substrate for the induced cytochrome P450, resulting in diminished inactive

Table 3.20 Influence of triacetyloleandomycin on hexobarbitone metabolism and sleeping time

Drug pretreatment	Hexobarbitone hydroxylase activity (nmol/min/mg)	Hexobarbitone sleeping time (min)
None	1.8 ± 0.7	22 ± 8
1 h after TAO,[a] 1 mmol/kg	1.7 ± 0.7	27 ± 9
24 h after TAO, 1 mmol/kg	1.2 ± 0.7	40 ± 18
TAO, 1 mmol/kg daily, for 4 days	0.3 ± 0.1	168 ± 58

[a] TAO; triacetyloleandomycin.
From Pessayre, D. et al. (1981), *Biochem. Pharmacol.* **30**, 559–564, with permission from Elsevier Science.

Table 3.21 Miscellaneous drugs and xenobiotics that inhibit drug metabolism

Drug/xenobiotic	Use or occurrence	Nature of inhibitory action
Amantadine	Anti-viral drug	Specific mode of action unknown, may alter synthesis or degradation of cytochrome P450.
7,8-Benzoflavone	Plant constituent	Complex action, relatively specific competitive inhibitor of cytochrome P4501A sub-family.
Carbon disulfide	Vulcanisation of rubber, intermediate in rayon manufacture, occupational exposure significant	Denaturation and loss of hepatic cytochrome P450, sulfur binding to microsomal proteins possibly induces lipid peroxidation.
Carbon tetrachloride	Solvent	Loss of liver microsomal enzymes, lipid peroxidation, activated by cytochrome P450-dependent metabolism (carbon–halogen bond cleavage).
Cimetidine	Anti-ulcer drug	Binds to cytochrome P450 (competitive inhibitor?)
Chloramphenicol	Broad spectrum antibiotic	Competitive inhibitor of cytochrome P450, also non-competitive inhibition due to covalent binding to apoenzyme of cytochrome P450 (suicide substrate).
Cyclophosphamide	Anti-cancer and immunosuppressant drug	Denaturation of cytochrome P450 by alkylation of sulfhydryl groups in active site.
Disulfiram	Therapy of alcoholics	Blocks ethanol oxidation at stage of acetaldehyde by inhibiting aldehyde oxidase.
Ellipticine	Anti-cancer drug	Potent competitive inhibitor of cytochrome P4501A sub-family.
Indomethacin	Anti-inflammatory drug	Depletes cytochrome P450 by unknown mechanism.
MAO inhibitors	Anti-depressant drugs	Inhibits monoamine oxidase (MAO) and enzymes of drug metabolism.
Metyrapone	Diagnosis of pituitary function	Binds tightly to and inhibits cytochrome P450.
Parathion	Insecticide	Haem loss and binding of atomic sulfur to cytochrome P450.
Tilorone	Anti-viral agent (interferon inducer)	Alters cytochrome P450 turnover, probably by increasing its degradation, or inhibition of synthesis.

From Pessayre et al. (1981) Biochem. Pharmacol., **30**, 559–564, with permission from Elsevier Science.

cytochrome P450 complex formation. This reduced activity of oleandomycin is consistent with the observation that no severe drug–drug interactions have been reported in man and indicates that oleandomycin may be a safer substitute for triacetyloleandomycin in patients who receive other drugs metabolised by cytochrome P450.

3.3.5 Inhibition of drug metabolism: miscellaneous drugs and xenobiotics

The inhibition of drug metabolism is by no means confined to the above groups of compounds and, as shown in Table 3.21, many drugs and xenobiotics of diverse chemical structure can act through a variety of mechanisms to decrease the biotransformation of drugs. Again, the liver appears to be the most important and susceptible target organ for inhibition of drug metabolism and the examples given in Table 3.21 are only representative of the many reported instances of decreased drug metabolism.

It is also of relevance here to note that the drug-metabolising enzymes are also regulated by 'internal factors' involving endogenous or constitutive mechanisms. For example, interferons and interleukin cytokines produced by viral infections can lead to a down-regulation of cytochrome P450 mRNA at the transcriptional level. In addition, the activity of the cytochrome P450 enzymes is substantially reduced by cAMP-dependent protein kinases and phosphorlyation of serine residues. This short-term regulation of the cytochromes P450 is thought to arise from phosphorylation-dependent destruction of the cytochromes P450, some enzymes being more susceptible to destruction than others. This general concept of internal factors regulating drug metabolism is dealt with in much more detail in the next chapter.

3.4 BIOLOGICAL SIGNIFICANCE OF INDUCTION AND INHIBITION OF DRUG METABOLISM

3.4.1 Drug tolerance

It has long been recognised that patients develop tolerance to the continued use of barbiturates and this is a consequence of the barbiturates inducing the cytochromes P450 that metabolise the drugs. Hence, on chronic exposure, the blood levels of barbiturates drop and the dose needs to be increased to sustain sedation, i.e. the development of tolerance.

3.4.2 Variability in drug response

In man, excessive drinking of alcohol and heavy smoking result in induction of several cytochromes P450 involved in drug metabolism. Accordingly, these population sub-groups have an increased ability to metabolise drugs and it is not uncommon for them to exhibit therapeutic failure in the clinical setting, as these lifestyle habits are largely ignored in prescribing drugs. More often than not, this effective resistance to drugs can be overcome by increasing the dose.

3.4.3 Drug–drug interactions and clinical pharmacology

The diverse range of substrates, inducers and inhibitors of the cytochromes P450 creates the potential for clinically significant drug interactions, particularly in therapeutic areas where polypharmacy is common practice, for example in the elderly or in the long-term prophylaxis of psychiatric disorders. Whereas it is recognised that not every drug–drug interaction involving induction or inhibition of cytochrome P450-mediated metabolism results in altered clinical responses, there are sufficient reports in the literature where this is indeed the case. For example, cyclosporine (a drug used to prevent organ rejection after transplantation) is a CYP3A4 substrate and co-administration of the antibiotic rifampicin (a CYP3A4 inducer) has resulted in clinically defined organ graft rejection. Thus, variation in the expression of the cytochromes P450 can therefore impact on substantial variation in the clinical usage (first-pass metabolism) and potential toxicity of drug–drug interactions in man.

Enzyme inhibition can also result in drug–drug interactions and several well-characterised clinical problems have arisen in man. Examples of these inhibitors are cimetidine, gestodene and terfenadine. The latter compound is extensively metabolised by CYP3A4 to such an extent that hardly any parent drug is found in plasma. Terfenadine was initially very successful as it was the first non-sedating antihistamine on the market but it has recently been withdrawn because of interactions with inhibitors such as ketoconazole, resulting in exaggerated plasma levels of the free drug which produced cardiac arrythmias.

Because of the large number of substrates, inhibitors and inducers of human cytochromes P450 (and other drug-metabolising enzymes), there is clearly a significant potential for drug–drug interactions with the subsequent alteration in therapeutic effectiveness, a concept to be developed more comprehensively in Chapter 7.

3.4.4 Drug and chemical toxicity

Tissue-specific expression of multiple forms of cytochrome P450 may provide an explanation of why only certain tissues are susceptible to chemically dependent toxicity, and therefore induction/inhibition has the potential to alter toxicological responses to drugs and other xenobiotics. For example, many chemicals that are known to cause cancer in experimental animals are biologically inert *per se* and require metabolic oxidation by the cytochrome P450 enzyme system before they can ultimately express their carcinogenicity. An excellent example of the role of cytochrome P450 in the activation of innocuous chemicals to potent carcinogens is shown in Figure 3.9. In this example, inert benzo[a]pyrene (a ubiquitous environmental contaminant) is first metabolised by cytochrome P450 forming the 7,8-epoxide derivative which subsequently serves as the substrate for another microsomal enzyme, epoxide hydrolase, to form the 7,8-diol derivative of benzo[a]pyrene. This latter diol is further metabolised by cytochrome P450 to the potent, ultimate carcinogen, benzo[a]pyrene 7,8-diol-9,10-epoxide, which can

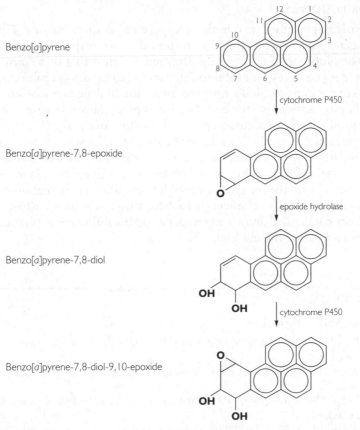

Benzo[a]pyrene

cytochrome P450

Benzo[a]pyrene-7,8-epoxide

epoxide hydrolase

Benzo[a]pyrene-7,8-diol

cytochrome P450

Benzo[a]pyrene-7,8-diol-9,10-epoxide

Figure 3.9 Role of cytochrome P450 in the activation of the procarcinogen, benzo[a]pyrene. The first epoxidation reaction is catalysed mainly by the CYP1A3 and the second by CYP3As and CYP1As.

then bind to nucleic acids and initiate the complex series of events leading to cancer. Therefore it is clear that any tissue that contains the appropriate cytochrome P450 enzymes (CYPs 1A and 3A) to catalyse the two oxidation reactions in Figure 3.9 (and, of course, epoxide hydrolase) may be susceptible to carcinogenesis by this chemical, particularly if the tissue levels are high as a result of prior enzyme induction. In reality, the biological situation is much more complex than outlined above and other factors, including, for example, the role of detoxifying, conjugating (phase 2) enzymes and the role of DNA repair mechanisms, are important in determining tissue susceptibility to chemical carcinogens. However, it is clear from the above considerations that cytochrome P450 has a substantial role to play in chemical carcinogenesis, and susceptibility to enzyme induction can exacerbate the toxic response. The interested reader is referred to Chapter 6 for a fuller discussion of this phenomenon.

3.5 CONCLUSIONS

The study of drug metabolism is both a complex and challenging one. This chapter has highlighted some of the chemical factors that are responsible for either the induction or inhibition of drug metabolism, and it is clear that these factors make a significant and complex contribution to modulating drug biotransformation. Awareness of the extent of induction and inhibition of drug metabolism is complicated by the observation that the body burden of potentially regulatory chemicals is unknown to any degree of accuracy, primarily because of the significant role played by environmental chemicals. Because of the variable exposure of man to pharmaceutical products and environmental chemicals, it is not absolutely certain that we can define 'basal levels' of drug metabolism in any given population or ethnic group. However, with the refinement of epidemiological and animal/human studies in drug metabolism, we can confidently look forward to the future when at least we will have fully catalogued and largely understood the influence of pharmaceuticals and chemicals on drug metabolism.

FURTHER READING

Textbooks and symposia

Burris, T.P. and McCabe, M. (2001) *Nuclear Receptors and Genetic Disease*. Academic Press, San Diego.

Ioannides, C. (1996) *Cytochromes P450: Metabolic and Toxicological Aspects*. CRC Press, Boca Raton, FL.

Lewis, D.F.V. (1996) *Cytochromes P450: Structure, Function and Mechanism*. Taylor and Francis, London.

Ruckpaul, K. and Rein, H. (eds) (1990) *Frontiers in Biotransformation, vol. 2: Principles, Mechanisms and Biological Consequences of Induction*. Taylor and Francis, London.

Stockley, I.H. (1996) *Drug Interactions*, 4th edn. The Pharmaceutical Press, London.

Woolf, T.F. (ed.) (1999) *Handbook of Drug Metabolism*. Marcel Dekker, New York.

Xenobiotica. Special Issue on Human Cytochrome P450s. (1998) 28 (12), 1095–1273.

Reviews and original articles

Boobis, A.R. *et al.* (1990) Species variation in the response of the cytochrome P450-dependent monooxygenase system to inducers and inhibitors. *Xenobiotica* 20, 39–61.

Bradfield, C.A. *et al.* (1991) Purification and N-terminal amino acid sequence of the Ah receptor from the C57BL/6J mouse. *Molec. Pharmacol.* 39, 13–19.

Burbach, K.M. *et al.* (1992) Cloning of the Ah receptor cDNA reveals a distinctive ligand-activated transcription factor. *Proc. Nat. Acad. Sci. USA* 89, 185–189.

Chen, Y.L. *et al.* (1992) Effects of interleukin-6 on cytochrome P450-dependent mixed function oxidases in the rat. *Biochem. Pharmacol.* 44, 137–148.

Clarke, S.E. (1998) *In vitro* assessment of human cytochrome P450. *Xenobiotica* 28, 1167–1202.

Corton, J.C. *et al.* (2000) Central role of peroxisome proliferator receptors in the actions of peroxisome proliferators. *Ann. Rev. Pharmacol. Toxicol.* 40, 491–518.

Gibson, G.G. (1996) Peroxisome proliferators and cytochrome P4504A induction. In: *Peroxisomes: Biology and Role in Toxicology and Disease* (J.K. Reddy *et al.*, eds). *Ann. NY Acad. Sci.* **804**, 328–340.

Goodwin, B. *et al.* (1999) The orphan nuclear human pregnane X receptor mediates the transcriptional activation by rifampicin through a distal enhancer module. *Drug Metab. Disp.* **56**, 1329–1339.

Green, S. (1992) Commentary: receptor-mediated mechanisms of peroxisome proliferators. *Biochem. Pharmacol.* **43**, 393–401.

Guengerich, F.P. (1999a) Cytochrome P450 3A4: regulation and role in metabolism. *Ann. Rev. Pharmacol. Toxicol.* **39**, 1–17.

Guengerich, F.P. (1999b) Inhibition of drug-metabolising enzymes: molecular and biochemical aspects. In: *Handbook of Drug Metabolism* (T.F. Woolf, ed.). Marcel Dekker, New York, pp 203–227.

Hankinson, O. *et al.* (1991) Genetic and molecular analysis of the Ah receptor and CYPIAI gene expression. *Biochimie* **73**, 61–66.

Hashimoto, H. *et al.* (1993) Gene structure of CYP3A4, an adult-specific cytochrome P450 in human livers, and its transcriptional control. *Eur. J. Biochem.* **218**, 585–595.

Honkakoski, P. and Negishi, M. (2000) Regulation of cytochrome P450 genes by nuclear receptors. *Biochem. J.* **347**, 321–337.

Hooper, W.D. (1999) Metabolic drug interactions. In: *Handbook of Drug Metabolism* (T.F. Woolf, ed.). Marcel Dekker, New York, pp 229–238.

Issemann, I. and Green, S. (1990) Activation of a member of the steroid hormone receptor superfamily by peroxisome proliferators. *Nature* **347**, 645–650.

Jones, S.A. *et al.* (2000) The pregnane X receptor: a promiscuous xenobiotic receptor that has diverged during evolution. *Molec. Endocrinol.* **14**, 27–39.

Moore, L.B. *et al.* (2000) The orphan nuclear receptors, constitutive androstane receptor and pregnane X receptor share xenobiotic and steroid ligands. *J. Biol. Chem.* **275**, 15 122–15 127.

Morgan, E.T. (2001) Minireview. Regulation of cytochrome P450 by inflammatory mediators: why and how. *Drug Metab. Disp.* **29**, 207–212.

Murray, M. (1992) P450 enzymes: inhibition mechanisms, genetic regulation and effects of liver disease. *Clin. Pharmacokin.* **23**, 132–146.

Park, B.K. and Kitteringham, N.R. (1990) Assessment of enzyme induction and enzyme inhibition in humans: toxicological implications. *Xenobiotica* **20**, 1171–1185.

Pascussi, J.M. *et al.* (2000) Dexamethasone induces pregnane X receptor and retinoid X receptor expression in human hepatocytes: synergistic increase of CYP3A4 induction by pregnane X receptor activators. *Molec. Pharmacol.* **58**, 361–362.

Pelkonen, O. *et al.* (1998) Inhibition and induction of human cytochrome P450 enzymes. *Xenobiotica* **28**, 1203–1253.

Ronis, M.J.J. and Ingelman-Sundberg, M. (1999) Induction of human drug-metabolising enzymes: mechanisms and implications. In: *Handbook of Drug Metabolism* (T.F. Woolf, ed.). Marcel Dekker, New York, pp 239–262.

Scheutz, E.G. *et al.* (2000) The glucocorticoid receptor is essential for induction of cytochrome P450 2B by steroids, but not for drug or steroid induction of CYP3A or P450 reductase in mouse liver. *Drug Metab. Disp.* **28**, 268–278.

Smith, D.A. *et al.* (1998) Human cytochromes P450: selectivity and measurement in vivo. *Xenobiotica* **28**, 1095–1128.

Smith, G. *et al.* (1998) Molecular genetics of the human cytochrome P450 monooxygenase superfamily. *Xenobiotica* **28**, 1129–1165.

Sueyoshi, T. *et al.* (1999) The repressed nuclear receptor CAR responds to phenobarbital in activating the human CYP2B6 gene. *J. Biol. Chem.* **274**, 6043–6046.

Testa, B. (1990) Mechanisms of inhibition of xenobiotic-metabolising enzymes. *Xenobiotica* **20**, 1129–1137.

Thummel, K.E. and Wilkinson, G.R. (1998) *In vitro* and *in vivo* drug interactions involving human CYP3A. *Ann. Rev. Pharmacol. Toxicol.* **38**, 389–430.

Wang, R.W. *et al.* (2000) Human cytochrome P450 3A4: *in vitro* drug–drug interaction patterns are substrate-dependent. *Drug Metab. Disp.* **28**, 360–366.

Waxman, D.J. (1999) P450 gene induction by structurally diverse xenochemicals: central role of nuclear receptors CAR, PXR and PPAR. *Arch. Biochem. Biophys.* **369**, 11–23.

Werk-Reichart, D. and Feyereisen, R. (2000) Cytochrome P450: a success story. *Genome Biol.* **1**, 1–9.

Whitlock, J.P. (1999) Induction of CYP1A1. *Ann. Rev. Pharmacol. Toxicol.* **39**, 103–125.

Wrighton, S. *et al.* (2000) The human CYP3A subfamily: practical considerations. *Drug Metab. Rev.* **32**, 339–361.

Xie, W. *et al.* (2000) Humanised xenobiotic response in mice expressing nuclear receptor SXR. *Nature* **406**, 435–439.

Web sites

- Directory of P450-containing systems (updates on P450 sequences).
  http://base.icgeb.trieste.it/p450/
- Cytochrome P450: a wealth of information on P450 structure (and related redox proteins), steroid ligands of P450s, selected references on P450-containing systems, families of structural domains of P450-containing systems, structural domains of P450-containing systems, images of known P450 3D structures, table of age-dependent changes in liver microsomal P450 and a tree of representative P450 sequences.
  http://www.icgeb.trieste.it/~p450srv/
- Human Cytochrome P450 Allele Nomenclature Committee.
  http://www.imm.ki.se/CYPalleles/
- Human P450 Metabolism Data Base. A very user-friendly site that gives a wealth of information on P450 multiple forms, drug substrates and inducers/inhibitors of CYPs (all categories with representative literature reference).
  http://www.gentest.com/human_p450_database/index.html

4 FACTORS AFFECTING DRUG METABOLISM: INTERNAL FACTORS

LEARNING OBJECTIVES

At the end of this chapter, you should be able to:
- Discuss, using named examples and giving mechanisms, how the genetic make-up, age, sex or hormonal status of the animal or person can affect the rate and pathways of metabolism of drugs
- Discuss, using named examples and giving mechanisms, how disease states may affect the rate and pathways of metabolism of drugs
- Assess how the above factors may affect the intensity, duration of action and toxicity of drugs through alterations in metabolism

---

4.1 INTRODUCTION

Drugs can be metabolised by many different pathways (see Chapter 1) and many factors can determine which pathway is used by which drug and to what extent a particular drug is biotransformed by a particular pathway. These factors range from the species of organism studied to the environment in which that organism lives. In order to discuss this topic, the factors affecting drug metabolism will be split into internal (i.e. physiological and pathological) factors (discussed in this chapter) and external factors (i.e. diet and environment) (discussed in Chapter 5). These are, of course, purely arbitrary divisions and much interaction exists between the various factors (cf. hormonal, sex and age influences) – such interactions will be pointed out where they are important. The factors discussed here are also not an exhaustive list and other factors that play a role in controlling drug biotransformation will be found in the further reading section at the end of Chapter 5. The factors to be discussed here are listed below:

INTERNAL: species, genetic, age, sex, hormones, disease
EXTERNAL: diet and environment

Each of these factors will be examined in turn, giving examples of the differences seen.

4.2 SPECIES DIFFERENCES

Species differences in drug/xenobiotic metabolism have been known for many years but have become topical due to the necessity to relate metabolism of drugs in animal systems to that in man during routine drug testing and the advent of simpler test systems (e.g. isolated liver cells) which allow a closer investigation of interspecies variability. These systems and their uses will be discussed further in

Table 4.1 The species variation in hexobarbitone metabolism, half-life and sleeping time

	Sleeping time (min)	Hexobarbitone half-life (min)	Hexobarbitone metabolism (units)
Mice	12 ± 8^a	19 ± 7	16.6
Rats	90 ± 15	140 ± 54	3.7
Dog	315 ± 105	260 ± 20	1
Man		~360	

[a] Mean ± (standard deviation)
(Data from Quinn, G.P. et al. (1958) Biochem. Pharmacol. 1, 152–159. Reprinted with permission of Pergamon Press.)

Chapter 7. Species differences can be found for both phase 1 and phase 2 metabolism and can be either quantitative (same metabolic route but differing rates) or qualitative (differing metabolic routes). Some examples of each of these cases are given below.

Very early data (shown in Table 4.1) indicated that the overall oxidative metabolism of hexobarbitone varies widely between species and is inversely related to the half-life and duration of action of the drug. This direct relationship between metabolism, half-life and action of a drug, however, does not always hold true. These problems are further discussed in Chapter 7. In this case, however, this would seem to indicate that man metabolises hexobarbitone at a slower rate than the dog and that the rate of elimination of the drug from the body is dependent on the metabolism of the drug. Other species differences in phase 1 metabolism can be seen for caffeine (Table 4.2) where the formation of paraxanthine is highest in man and lowest in monkey, whereas theophylline production is highest in monkey and lowest in man. Further examples coming to light using isolated whole liver preparations include the marked species differences in thiabendazole (an anthelminthic) metabolism with the rabbit hepatocytes producing 5-hydroxythiabendazole at a rate over 40 times that of comparable rat cells. As can be seen from Figure 4.1 oxyphenbutazone is rapidly cleared in the dog ($T_{1/2}$ 30 min) whilst, in man, the rate of metabolism is rather slow ($T_{1/2}$ 3 days). This is an extreme example but clearly indicates the possible range of species differences.

In terms of phase 2 metabolism, sulfadimethoxine is converted to the glucuronide in man but no glucuronide formation is evident in rat, guinea pig or rabbit. Phenol is metabolised by conjugation to glucuronic acid and/or sulfate and the

Table 4.2 Species differences in caffeine metabolism

Parameter	Man	Monkey	Rat	Rabbit
Total metabolism	322	235	160	137
Theobromine	28	13	15	19
Paraxanthine	193	11	20	42
Theophylline	16	190	20	30

Results expressed as pmoles of product per min.mg protein.
Data taken from Berthou F. et al. (1992) Xenobiotica 22, 671–680.

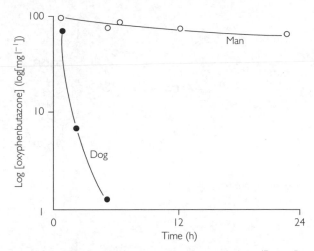

Figure 4.1 Plasma levels of oxyphenobutazone in man and dog. (From Burns, J.J. (1962) In: *Metabolic Factors Controlling Duration of Drug Action* (B.B. Brodie and E.G. Erdos, eds). Pergamon, Oxford, p. 278.

relative proportion of each metabolite depends on the species studied (Table 4.3). The detoxification of trichloroethylene, a widespread environmental contaminant, by conjugation to glutathione is also known to be species dependent. Mouse kidney is over 12 times better at detoxifying trichloroethylene than the same tissue in rats, whereas mouse liver is only 2–4 times better than the comparable tissue in rats.

All the above are simple examples of one or two enzymes acting on one compound. The situation can, however, become quite complex when a larger number of reactions are involved in the metabolism of one compound. Such a compound is amphetamine, the overall metabolism of which is shown in Figure 4.2.

The rat mainly hydroxylates amphetamine, leading to conjugated products on the phenol group, whereas the rabbit and guinea pig (and man) mainly deaminate amphetamine. The guinea pig further oxidises the ketone to benzoic acid and excretes conjugates of benzoic acid. The rabbit has been shown to reduce the ketone and excrete the subsequent conjugates of the alcohol.

Table 4.3 The species variation in the relative proportions of phenol conjugation to glucuronide and sulfate

	Phenol conjugation[a]	
	Glucuronide	**Sulfate**
Cat	0	87
Man	23	71
Rat	25	68
Rabbit	46	45
Pig	100	0

[a] Expressed as excretion of a particular conjugate as a percentage of total excretion of drug.
(Data from various sources; see further reading section in Chapter 5.)

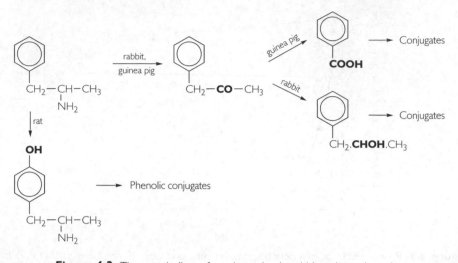

Figure 4.2 The metabolism of amphetamine in rabbit, guinea pig and rat.

It is clear that different species can differ in their routes of metabolism as well as in the rates at which the metabolism occurs. Many other species have now been tested for drug metabolising ability such as farm species (sheep, goats, cattle), fish, birds and even microorganisms and plants. In general, drug metabolism in non-mammalian species is lower than in mammals. Species differences in drug metabolism are important to industries involved in testing new chemicals in order to achieve a suitable model of human toxicity. For such purposes an animal model is required that mimics as closely as possible the metabolism of the compound seen in man. This animal model may be different for the different compounds under study.

4.3 GENETIC DIFFERENCES

It has been noted above that significant differences in drug metabolism are found between species – it is equally true, however, that such differences exist within species. This is most easily seen in the inbred populations of rats and mice used in many studies but is also being found for other species, including man. Such differences are referred to as genetic polymorphism.

The classical example of strain differences in drug metabolism is that of hexobarbitone metabolism in the mouse (see Table 4.4). There is up to a 2.5-fold difference in sleeping time between one strain of mouse and another and the values for the animals in the inbred groups are close to each other whereas the outbred group shows a wide variation in sleeping time. This is clear evidence for a genetic control of drug metabolism. The marked strain differences in the mouse have also been extended to include differences in the induction of drug metabolism (see Chapter 3). Using two strains of mouse it was shown that one (strain C57) responds

Strain	Sleeping time (min)
A/NL	48 ± 4^a
BALB/cAnN	41 ± 2
C57L/HeN	33 ± 3
C3HFB/HeN	22 ± 3
SWR/HeN	18 ± 4
Swiss (outbred)	43 ± 15

Table 4.4 Hexobarbitone sleeping time in various strains of mouse

[a] Mean $\pm$ (standard deviation)
All animals were age-matched males and were given a standard dose of hexobarbitone.
(Data from various sources; see further reading section in Chapter 5.)

to treatment with 3-methylcholanthrene (3-MC, a polycyclic hydrocarbon inducer of aryl hydrocarbon hydroxylase) whilst the other (strain DBA) does not. Cross breeding of the strains (see Table 4.5) has shown that the inheritance of inducibility is an autosomal dominant (Ah^d) trait and accounted for by the presence of the Ah receptor. The biochemical mechanism of this induction is discussed in Chapter 3.

In the rat, strain differences are reported to be less common and have centred mainly around the genetically deficient Gunn rat, which is unable to form many of the glucuronides produced by other strains of rats. Interbreeding of Gunn and normal rat strains leads to glucuronidation capacities intermediate between the two, indicating that neither trait is dominant.

In man the possibility of showing a pure genetic influence on drug metabolism is hampered by interfering influences from environmental sources as it is impossible to keep humans in controlled conditions of environment, diet, etc., during their lifespan. It has, however, been possible to show probable genetic effects on drug metabolism that have subsequently been proved using molecular biological techniques.

It has been recognised for a long time that large variations in drug metabolism occur in man and that discrete genetic sub-populations are present in the human population. One such sub-population is the group of 'isoniazid slow acetylators'.

Strain	% Inducible
C57 (Ah^dAh^d)[a]	100
DBA (Ah^bAh^b)[a]	0
F1 (C57 × DBA) (Ah^bAh^d)[a]	100
F1 × C57	100
F1 × DBA	50
F1 × F1	75

Table 4.5 Effect of cross-breeding on the inducibility of polycyclic hydrocarbons of aryl hydrocarbon hydroxylase in mice

[a] Ah is the gene for inducibility for polycyclic hydrocarbons. Ah^d, inducible; Ah^b, not inducible
(Data from various sources; see further reading section in Chapter 5.)

The acetylation of isoniazid in the human population exhibits a bimodal distribution, with about half the Caucasian population 'fast acetylators' and half 'slow acetylators'. Family studies show that 'slow acetylation' is an autosomal recessive trait. The unusually high incidence of this recessive trait in the population indicates that 'slow acetylation' must confer some sort of advantage or be closely linked to a gene giving such an advantage.

A similar problem to the Gunn rat is seen in man with decreased ability to glucuronidate bilirubin, leading to Crigler–Najjar syndrome or the less severe Gilbert's Disease.

With respect to phase 1 metabolism by cytochrome P450, it has long been thought that some sort of genetic control was in operation based on the 'twin' studies of Vessell and others. It was found that identical twins resembled each other very closely in terms of drug metabolism whereas fraternal twins (twins developed from two different eggs) showed variations similar to the general population. Also the rates of metabolism of desmethylimipramine, nortriptyline, phenylbutazone and dicoumarol show good mutual correlation, indicating a common mechanism of control of their metabolism. Extensive studies using the marker substrate debrisoquine have shown a definite genetic polymorphism in CYP2D6-dependent drug oxidation. The 4-hydroxylation of this compound shows a bimodal distribution in the population. Again twin, family and population studies have indicated that the 'poor metaboliser' (PM) trait is recessive. In this case, however, no advantage appears to be linked to the PM trait as these are in low frequency in the population. The metabolism of a number of other drugs has now been linked to debrisoquine 4-hydroxylation so that poor metabolisers of debrisoquine also show low metabolism of sparteine, amitriptyline, phenformin, haloperidol and phenacetin, amongst others. A simple test (debrisoquine 4-hydroxylation) could therefore be used to pinpoint patients at risk due to low metabolism of the drug to be administered. Other individual differences in oxidative drug metabolism do not correlate to debrisoquine metabolism and may represent other genes controlling cytochrome P450, such as that for the metabolism of dextromethorphan and mephenytoin 4-hydroxylation. These polymorphisms are becoming regarded as of great clinical significance and have spawned the expanding field of pharmaco-genetics – a topic to be discussed in greater detail in Chapter 7.

Another aspect of genetic control of drug metabolism is the appearance of racial differences. Differences between the metabolism of propranolol in Negro and Caucasian populations exist as do differences in the glucuronidation of paracetamol between Caucasians and Chinese. Clear indications of the genetic nature of these differences has again come from molecular biology with differences noted in the genes for CYP2D6 and CYP2C9 (amongst others) in Polynesians of the South Pacific and Japanese, respectively. African and Afro-American populations have also been shown to have genetic differences in drug metabolism.

Genetic differences within a population can affect the rate at which drugs are metabolised and there is convincing evidence to support a direct genetic control of some oxidative and conjugative reactions.

4.3.1 Mechanisms of control of species and genetic differences

The use of powerful molecular biological techniques has shown that most species and genetic differences in drug metabolism arise because of the presence of genes coding for different enzymes. The inability of the cat to glucuronidate phenol is due to the absence of a phenol glucuronosyltransferase, whereas the bilirubin glucuronosyltransferase is still present, allowing the cat to clear the endogenous compound, bilirubin. The Gunn rat is deficient in a number of glucuronosyl-transferase activities and also has defective glucuronosyltransferase genes. A number of defective genes have been detected and isolated from the Gunn rat. Both Crigler–Najjar Syndrome and Gilbert's Disease in man have been shown to be defects in the UGT1A1 gene. The species and strain differences in glucuronidation are thus due to the presence of different enzyme forms that in turn are the products of different (and sometimes defective) genes. This is also the case for the 'fast' and 'slow' acetylators. The abnormality has been traced to a defective gene both in the rat and in man.

Species differences in phase 1 oxidative metabolism are also thought to be based on the different complement of cytochrome P450 in the different species. Around 800 different forms of cytochrome P450 are now recognised, some having widespread distribution (e.g. forms 1A1 and 2E1) whereas others appear to be found only in one species (e.g. the human-specific 2B7). The complement of cytochrome P450 forms determines, therefore, the range of oxidative processes seen for individual drugs. A recent review by Guengerich (1997) has correlated the detection of various forms of cytochrome P450 with specific enzyme activities in different species. For a further discussion of forms of drug-metabolising enzymes and their nomenclature, see Chapter 2.

A great deal of research has been performed on the polymorphism of cytochrome P450, particularly related to debrisoquine hydroxylation and it has been found that one form of cytochrome P450 (CYP2D6) is responsible for this enzyme activity in man. In the 'poor metaboliser' phenotype this form was absent from the liver and at least three mutant alleles of the CYP2D6 gene have been identified in 'poor metabolisers'. Indeed, a large array of mutations have been identified using molecular biological techniques, some of which have little effect on activity of the enzyme product whereas others reduce or increase enzyme activity while some cause a virtually complete failure of enzyme production (so-called null mutations). One such example is given in Figure 4.3 where it is seen that a single point mutation

DNA	TCCG GTGG ... CCAG GACGCCC	TCCG GTGG ... CCAAG ACGCCCC
mRNA	UCC GGA CGC ... UGA (498 STOP)	UCC GAC GCC ... UGA (182 STOP)
Protein	Ser Gly Arg (497 amino acids)	Ser Asp Ala (181 amino acids)

Figure 4.3 The effect of a single mutation at position 1934 in the CYP2D6 gene (seen in CYP2D6*4) on the subsequent protein product of the gene. The boxed sequences are the ends of exons 3 and 4. The position of the STOP codon (UGA) is given as a number after STOP.

Table 4.6 Polymorphic forms of CYP2D6. The actual mutation is shown as the nucleotide that changes (and its position) and what it changes to (e.g. $G_{1749}C$ indicates a change from G to C at position 1749). (Data taken from Smith *et al.* (1998) *Xenobiotica* **28**, 1129–1165.)

Allele name	Mutation	Effect on enzyme activity
CYP2D6*1	None	None
CYP2D6*2a	$G_{1749}C$; $C_{2938}T$; $G_{4268}C$	None
CYP2D6*3	A_{2367} deleted	Inactive
CYP2D6*4	$C_{188}T$; $C_{1062}A$; $A_{1072}G$	Inactive
CYP2D6*5	CYP2D6 deleted	Inactive
CYP2D6*6	T_{1795} deleted; $G_{2064}A$	Inactive
CYP2D6*7	$A_{3023}C$	Inactive
CYP2D6*8	$G_{1749}C$; $G_{1846}T$; $G_{2938}T$	Inactive
CYP2D6*9	A_{2703}, G_{2704}, A_{2705} deleted	Reduced
CYP2D6*10	$C_{188}T$; $C_{1127}T$; $G_{4268}C$	Reduced
CYP2D6*11	$G_{971}C$; $C_{1062}A$; $A_{1072}G$; $C_{1085}G$	Reduced

leads to premature termination of the protein sequence, thus explaining the lack of an immunoreactive CYP2D6 protein in these individuals. Further examples of mutations in the CYP2D6 gene and their effects on enzyme production and activity are given in Table 4.6.

Similar gene changes are also seen for the mephenytoin polymorphism that is correlated with alterations in activity of CYP2C19. The use of reverse transcription and amplification of mRNA from an individual with low S-mephenytoin 4′-hydroxylation has shown a 40 base pair deletion in exon 5. Such a deletion leads to premature termination of the protein sequence similar to that seen for some of the mutations of the CYP2D6 gene.

Polymorphisms have also been detected for the CYP1A1, CYP2A6, CYP2C9 and CYP2E1 genes. In the case of the CYP1A1 polymorphism, this can manifest itself as an increase in inducibility (mutation in the 3′-non-coding region of the gene) or an increased enzyme activity (an A to G nucleotide substitution at position 4889 leading to a isoleucine to valine substitution in the protein sequence).

In one instance at least, however, differences in the enzyme are not responsible for a species difference: this is the inability of dog liver to acetylate sulfonamides

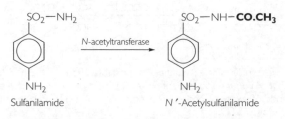

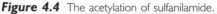

Figure 4.4 The acetylation of sulfanilamide.

(Figure 4.4). It has been suggested that a reversing enzyme, a deacetylase, converts the acetyl derivative back to the original compound or that a natural inhibitor exists in the dog.

4.4 AGE

It has long been recognised that the young, and particularly the newborn, and the old of many animals are more susceptible to drug action. Studies on the development of drug-metabolising capacity have indicated that this increased sensitivity of neonates may be related to their very low or, at times, unmeasurable drug-metabolising capacity which subsequently develops in a species-, strain-, substrate- and sex-dependent manner until adult levels of enzyme activity are achieved. The decrease in drug-metabolising capacity in old age also appears to be dependent on these factors although other specific factors may be involved.

4.4.1 Development of phase 1 metabolism

The activity of phase 1 drug metabolism may develop in many different ways between birth and adulthood and, indeed, may start developing at different times during gestation. The pattern of development varies according to the species and sex of the animal and on the substrate being investigated (and, thus, the particular form being studied). A general idea of the patterns of development is shown in Figure 4.5.

In the rat, type A development is seen for many aromatic and aliphatic hydroxylation reactions, e.g. aniline 4-hydroxylation. Type B development is shown for some *N*-demethylation reactions but in the case of hydroxylation of methylbenzanthracene, type B development is followed for a time but then activity falls to a very low level. Type C development is seen for the hydroxylation of 4-methylcoumarin.

In the rat, the sex differences (see the next section) in drug metabolism exhibited by the adult confuse the developmental profile. Consider the 16α-hydroxylase acting on androst-4-ene-3,17-dione (Figure 4.6): the enzyme activity develops

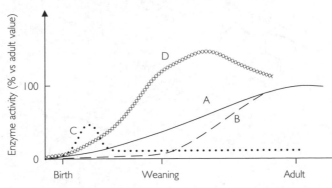

Figure 4.5 Developmental patterns for phase 1 metabolism. (From Sternberg, A. (1976) *J. Endocr.*, **68**, 265–72. Used with the permission of the author and publisher.)

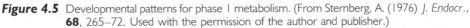

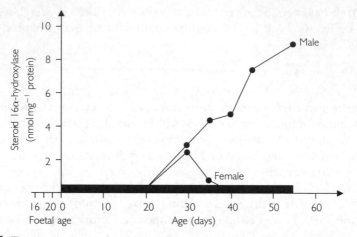

Figure 4.6 The development of the steroid 16α-hydroxylase in male and female rat liver. (From Sternberg, A. (1976) *J. Endocr.* **68**, 265–272. Used with the permission of the author and publisher.)

according to type B in both the male and the female but at 30 days of age (puberty in the female) the activity in the female begins to disappear and by 40 days of age is undetectable, thus giving the sex differences seen in the adult period.

In man and primates a somewhat different developmental profile is seen with measurable levels of activity in mid-term foetuses, indicating an earlier start to the process of development in primates. Indeed, some metabolic routes appear to be fully developed in foetal liver (e.g. the N-demethylation of codeine) whereas others are not present (e.g. O-demethylation of codeine)(Figure 4.7). Specific foetal forms of cytochrome P450 have been identified in man, such as CYP3A7,

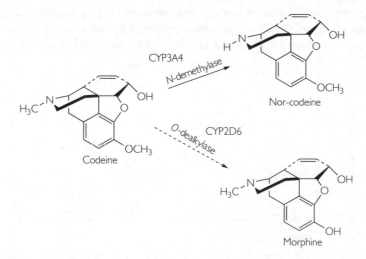

Figure 4.7 Two different metabolic routes for codeine.

that disappear at birth to be replaced by the adult forms, CYP3A4/5. It is, however, still quite clear that the foetus and neonate are, in general, less able to metabolise drugs than the adult.

In ageing animals and man, a further change in drug metabolism is seen. In rats a marked fall in overall drug-metabolising capacity is seen, e.g. for testosterone hydroxylation. These changes are, however, associated with the sex differences in drug metabolism seen in the rat (see the next section). There is evidence that the decline in drug metabolism in rats is also strain dependent. In man, it has been generally accepted that old age leads to a diminished capacity to clear drugs and evidence using probe substrates such as lignocaine, coumarin and antipyrine would seem to confirm this impression. In both men and women over 65–70 years of age, metabolism of these drugs is significantly decreased and this is correlated to a decrease in the relevant form of cytochrome P450.

Other phase 1 enzymes have been less well studied in terms of age-related changes in activity. The flavin monooxygenases in mouse liver have been shown to alter during early development with FMO1 and FMO5 being found in late foetuses (days 15–17) whereas FMO3 does not appear until 2 weeks post-partum. In man, FMO1 is found in foetal liver but FMO3 in adult liver.

4.4.2 Control of development of phase 1 metabolism

What are the biochemical changes associated with development of drug metabolising ability, and how are they controlled? These are two essential questions for our understanding of the ontogenesis of phase 1 metabolism.

Most work has been performed on the cytochrome P450-dependent oxidation of drugs in the rat liver and the changes noted were those associated with the components of the enzyme system, notably cytochrome P450 itself. The development of a particular metabolic pathway seems to be closely linked to the appearance of a functional form of cytochrome P450 associated with that particular enzyme activity. For example, the 7α-hydroxylation of testosterone is highest at 3 weeks of age and is associated with a rise in CYP2A1 (a form known to perform this reaction) whereas testosterone 16α-hydroxylation is associated with CYP2C11 and both of these are found to increase in parallel in male rats. The association between drug metabolism and cytochrome P450 form profile continues into old age with the male-specific cytochromes P450 (e.g. CYP2C11) decreasing, leading to a marked fall in the drug metabolising activities associated with these proteins. CYP3A2 is found at relatively high levels early in development (3 weeks) but has largely disappeared at 12–15 weeks of age in the rat.

The development of NADPH-cytochrome P450 reductase follows that of cytochrome P450 in most cases except that appreciable activity of this enzyme is found in newborn animals. In the rat and ferret, NADPH-cytochrome P450(c)-reductase is found in the neonatal period and the cytochrome P450 reductase does not develop until later. This cytochrome P450-reductase activity is thought to be associated with various azo reductase activities found in the neonatal period.

Hormonal changes during development can also have a profound effect on drug metabolism. The phenomenon of 'imprinting' of drug metabolism in the rat by

Table 4.7 The effect of reduced progesterone analogues on progesterone and coumarin metabolism in newborn rats

Progestagen added	Progesterone 16-hydroxylase	Coumarin 3-hydroxylase
None	24.1 ± 0.7[a]	5.0 ± 0.3
5β-Pregnane-3α,20α-diol	15.7 ± 0.7[a]	3.3 ± 0.4*
5β-Pregnane-3α-ol-20-one	15.5 ± 1.0*	2.3 ± 0.3*
5β-Pregnane-3,20-dione	16.8 ± 0.6*	3.1 ± 0.3*

[a] Activities expressed as nmoles metabolite formed per hour per mg protein; mean $\pm$ (standard deviation)
* = $p < 0.05$
(From Kordish, R. and Feuer, G. (1972) *Biol. Neonate* **20**, 50–67, modified. Used with permission of S. Karger AG, Basel.)

androgens, leading to sexual differentiation of enzyme activities in the adult period, is important in development. It is, in fact, thought that the rapid but transient increase in activity seen for some enzymes in the first few days after birth is due to the androgen secreted at this time in order to 'imprint' the male.

The rise in enzyme activity seen after weaning (type B development) is also thought to be hormone related – the hormone in this case being progesterone delivered to the infant in the mother's milk. Progestagens are, indeed, known to inhibit drug metabolism (see Table 4.7).

Growth hormone has also been shown to inhibit drug metabolism in the developing rat.

Even with all this wealth of information, the critical question: 'what is the rate-limiting step in the development of drug-metabolising capacity', remains unanswered. The answer is best summarised by Short who stated, 'It seems most likely that after birth the monooxygenase system develops largely as a unit'. The rate-limiting factor to the development of this unit depends on the species, strain and sex of the animal and the substrate under investigation.

4.4.3 Development of phase 2 metabolism

The development of phase 2 metabolism is of considerable importance as excretion of drugs and other xenobiotics is mainly in the form of conjugates – the conjugation reactions being generally regarded as the true 'detoxification' reactions. Changes in the ability of the body to conjugate drugs therefore leads to large changes in toxicity of the drugs. The balance between phase 1 and phase 2 metabolism during development is also of great importance. This topic will be further discussed in Chapter 6.

As with the phase 1 metabolism, phase 2 routes of metabolism are poorly represented in the foetal and neonatal animal and mainly develop perinatally.

4.4.3.1 Glucuronidation

The most thoroughly studied of the conjugation reactions is glucuronidation and here we are indebted to Professor G Dutton for his group's excellent work on the development of glucuronidation. This group has found that there are two different developmental types (not corresponding to the types found for phase 1 metabolism) as shown in Figure 4.8.

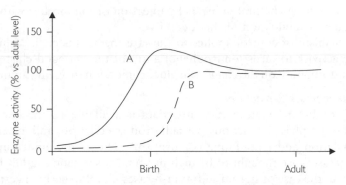

Figure 4.8 The developmental patterns of glucuronidation in the rat. Curve A is late foetal cluster (*p*-nitrophenol as substrate); B is neonatal cluster (bilirubin as substrate).

Type A development is characterised by a steadily increasing activity up until birth, reaching a peak around birth and then declining slightly to adult levels and type B development is characterised by very low activity until birth followed by a rapid rise to adult levels. Type A enzymes belong to the late foetal cluster of enzymes and metabolise predominantly exogenous compounds (e.g. *p*-nitrophenol) and type B belongs to the neonatal cluster of Greengard and metabolises mainly endogenous compounds (e.g. bilirubin). In man little glucuronidation activity is seen until after birth.

4.4.3.2 *Control of development of glucuronidation*
The appearance of glucuronosyltransferase activity during development appears to be closely linked to that of the glucuronosyltransferase protein.

The physiological control of development has been studied in some detail. One series of studies involved the use of chick embryos that can readily be cultured to facilitate the investigation. In this case, glucuronosyltransferase activity is negligible until hatching and then undergoes a rapid increase, reaching adult levels in 1–3 days. If embryonic liver is cultured its glucuronosyltransferase activity increases to adult levels spontaneously and precociously. The process of maturation involves a morphological change in the cells and protein synthesis. This precocious increase in activity in culture does not occur if the liver is cultured in the presence of the chorioallantoic membrane, indicating that induction of enzyme activity can only take place after removal of the repressive influence of the embryonic environment. The nature of this repressive influence is unclear. Certain hormones have, however, been shown to overcome this repressive influence such as corticosteroids (with thyroxine acting synergistically). In the chick, therefore, postnatal development is probably stimulated by corticosteroid production (and thyroxine).

In mammalian foetuses a similar mechanism of control has been shown to be in operation. Embryonic liver cultured on chorioallantoic membrane, as before, maintained its embryonic character. A pituitary graft onto the membrane stimulated glucuronosyltransferase activity to the adult level. Again, corticosteroids were shown to be the natural inducers by injection of the mother with hormones and subsequent examination of the foetal liver.

This mechanism of control applies to the late foetal cluster, i.e. glucuronosyl-transferase activity towards p-nitrophenol and not the neonatal cluster. There is little clear information on the changes in glucuronidation in ageing animals or man.

4.4.3.3 Other phase 2 reactions

Compared to glucuronidation very little data is available on the developmental patterns of other phase 2 reactions (i.e. sulfation, acetylation, amino acid conjugation, methylation and glutathione conjugation). The sulfo-conjugating enzymes (sulfotransferases) are thought to be high in foetal tissue (about adult levels) and, particularly in the case of steroid sulfotransferases, develop early in gestation. This is probably a function of their role in biosynthetic and transport pathways of metabolism rather than an excretory role. Growth hormones have been implicated in the control of development of steroid sulfotransferases (see the next section). An inhibitor of phenol sulfotransferases has also been found to be present at birth, accounting for the apparent fall in activity of the enzyme seen around this period.

For acetylation it was found that premature infants acetylate sulfonamides less well than full-term infants but this latter group are still below the activity of adults. In the rabbit, acetylation of isoniazid is low at 6 days, rises steadily to 14 days and then surges to adult levels between 21 and 28 days. In contrast, in the cow, N-acetylation of sulfamethoxazole is higher in the calf than the adult.

Amino acid conjugation and methylation are similar to acetylation, being low in foetal and neonatal tissues and developing steadily to adult levels.

Glutathione conjugation is of particular importance in being one of the major defence mechanisms in the body against electrophilic xenobiotics (many of which are mutagens and/or carcinogens). Early studies on the development of the enzyme responsible for glutathione conjugation (glutathione-S-transferase) showed a steady rise in activity from 3 days prenatally to 20 days postnatally in the rat by which time adult levels had been reached. In man an even earlier development of enzyme activity is thought to occur.

In summary, phase 2 metabolism is generally low or absent in foetal animals, develops perinatally, reaching adult levels early in life and does not seem to alter in any consistent way in old age. The multiplicity of the various enzymes involved should be remembered when studying these reactions in terms of development, as the different forms of the enzyme may develop at different times and different rates.

Age-related changes are seen by the clinician to be of major importance, as special dosage schedules for infants are used which are unrelated to the dose for an adult on a weight basis. The reduced metabolic activity of the older patients may also be important but this is of less general applicability.

4.5 HORMONAL CONTROL OF DRUG METABOLISM

Hormones play a major role in the control of drug metabolism and, in particular, the hormones of the pituitary, adrenal and testes are involved in this developmental control and sexual dimorphism. In this section it is intended to expand this idea to include all endocrine organs and to further examine the role of the pituitary, adrenal and sex glands and consider the thyroid and pancreas in terms of their effects on drug metabolism. The effects of pregnancy (as a major disturbance in the hormonal balance of the female body) on drug metabolism will also be discussed.

4.5.1 Pituitary gland

The pituitary gland controls the release of hormones from the other endocrine organs (except in the case of the pancreas where other influences are more important) and thus any effects exerted by the endocrine organs will be mimicked by the pituitary gland. Direct effects of pituitary hormones, such as growth hormones, have also been seen, however, as noted in Section 4.4. Other direct effects on hepatic drug metabolism are seen with adrenocorticotrophic hormone (ACTH), luteinizing hormone (LH), follicle-stimulating hormone (FSH) and prolactin. The pituitary gland, therefore, occupies a central role in the hormonal control of drug metabolism and the individual effects of this organ will be discussed under the various endocrine glands that it controls.

4.5.2 Sex glands

Sex glands in this context refer to the endocrine glands, the testes (in the male) producing androgens and the ovaries (in the female) producing estrogens and progestins. The effects of these hormones on drug metabolism are, as would be expected, mainly related to sex differences, although progestins (e.g. progesterone) have been implicated in the induction of CYP3A4 in women.

Sex differences in drug actions were first noted by Nicholas and Barron in 1932 who saw that female rats required only half the dose of barbiturate needed by male rats to induce sleep. Later studies indicated that this was due to the reduced capacity of the female to metabolise the barbiturates. Such sex differences in drug metabolism have now been shown for a wide range of substrates including the endogenous sex steroids. Sex differences in drug metabolism have also been noted in the mouse for ethylmorphine and steroid metabolism and in man for the pharmacokinetic parameters of clearance for a number of drugs, including antipyrine, diazepam and steroid hormones, although it is not clear how much of this difference is due to differences in metabolism as opposed to other pharmacokinetic factors (see Chapter 7). In general the sex differences seen in the mouse are the opposite of those seen in the rat whereas man shows a similar sex-differentiated pattern to the rat. Recently the goat has been shown to exhibit the opposite sex differences to those found in the rat.

Sex differences in the rat tend to follow a general pattern of the male metabolising faster than the female, particularly with regard to phase 1 metabolism, but there are exceptions, such as the 3-hydroxylation of lignocaine.

In phase 2 metabolism, there are marked sex differences in glucuronidation (e.g. of 1-naphthol), sulfation (e.g. of steroids) and glutathione conjugation, but again mainly in the rat. In the case of glucuronosyltransferases, the form metabolising 4-nitrophenol is found to be higher in the male whereas the estrone glucuronosyltransferase is higher in the female. For sulfotransferases, the aryl and nitrophenol sulfotransferase (SULT1) are higher in the male whereas the hydroxysteroid and bile acid sulfotransferasese (SULT20/21) are higher in the female.

4.5.3 Mechanism of control of sex differences

In 1958 it was proposed that androgens were the regulators of the sex differences. Thus the presence or absence of androgens in the perinatal period determines whether an animal is male or female with respect to drug metabolism – a process known as 'imprinting'. Although this still holds true, the mechanism by which perinatal androgens exert this effect is now well established and it is accepted that there is no direct effect of the androgen on the liver. The perinatal androgen

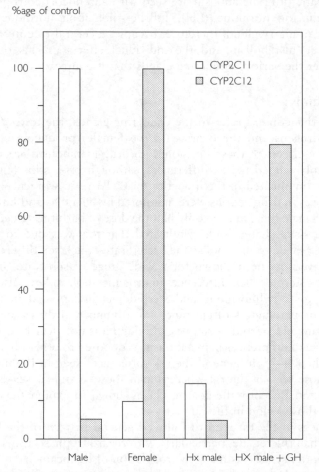

Figure 4.9 The effect of continuous growth hormone treatment on the expression of CYP2C11 and CYP2C12 genes. Hx = hypophysectomised.

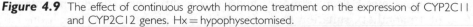

'imprints' a pattern of growth hormone secretion from the pituitary gland and it is this male or female pattern of growth hormone secretion that gives the sex differences in drug metabolism.

With respect to cytochrome P450-dependent drug oxidation, the differing patterns of growth hormone (GH) are known to cause the induction or repression of particular forms of cytochrome P450. For instance the female pattern of GH (a continuous low level of hormone) gives a reduction in CYP2C11 and an increase in CYP2C12 by altering the transcription of the particular gene. This alteration leads to the female type of metabolism – a decreased 16α-hydroxylase (associated with CYP2C11) and increased 15β-hydroxylase activity (associated with CYP2C12) (Figure 4.9).

Investigation of flavin monooxygenases in mouse liver has shown influences of androgens and estrogens in the whole animal on FMO1 and FMO3. More detailed work using isolated rat hepatocytes has shown a direct effect of 17β-estradiol on FMO activity but no effect of androgens or GH. The control of FMOs seems, thus, to be different to cytochrome P450-dependent monooxygenases.

In phase 2 metabolism, GH is also seen to be a controlling influence on glucuronosyltransferases (UGTs). Bilirubin glucuronidation is increased by hypophysectomy and returned to control levels by treatment with GH. These effects are seen to be related to changes in expression of the UGT1B1 and 1B2 genes. A similar dependence on GH is found for sulfotransferases with SULT1C1 (found in 10-fold higher concentrations in male rat liver and implicated in the activation of the carcinogen, N-hydroxyacetylaminofluorene) decreasing on hypophysectomy to the female level and being restored to male levels by intermittent treatment with GH.

Sex differences in drug metabolism are of great importance when dealing with rats, mice and some farm animals (e.g. goats) but seem to be of less importance in a clinical context.

4.5.4 Adrenal glands

The adrenal glands have already been discussed in terms of glucocorticoid control of development of drug metabolism (see Section 4.4). The adrenal glands are, however, also thought to be involved in the regulation of drug metabolism in the adult period. Adrenalectomy has been shown to reduce the phase 1 microsomal metabolism of a number of xenobiotics, whereas glucocorticoid replacement therapy can reverse the effect of adrenalectomy (see Figure 4.10).

Glucocorticoids have, however, been shown to mimic or potentiate the action of adrenalectomy in a number of instances. This apparent paradox in glucocorticoid action was resolved by Tredger who showed that the natural, short-acting glucocorticoids are inhibitory to drug metabolism whereas the synthetic potent analogues (which are not so readily metabolised) are stimulatory (act as enzyme inducers).

Few effects of adrenal hormones are seen on phase 2 metabolism except as regards development (see above) but again synthetic glucocorticoids (e.g. dexamethasone) can induce some phenol sulfotransferase activities and have an inhibitory effect on the expression of some glutathione-S-transferases (e.g. GSTP1).

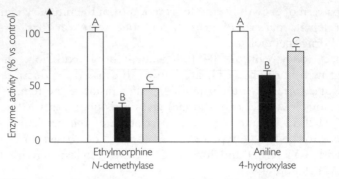

4.5.5 Thyroid gland

The thyroid gland is known to have some influence on drug metabolism. The effect of thyroidectomy in the rat depends on the substrate being studied and on the sex of the animal used (see Table 4.8).

In a study of the phase 1 metabolism of lignocaine, it was shown that there was an increase in the N-deethylation and 3-hydroxylation in both male and female animals whereas imipramine and diazepam metabolism were unaffected in the male. Imipramine metabolism was enhanced in the female. The effects noted in the earlier studies could be reversed by L-thyroxine treatment.

In the human, the thyroid gland has also been implicated in the control of drug metabolism. For the limited number of substrates used (antipyrine, paracetamol and aspirin), thyroidectomy always decreases their apparent metabolism.

The mechanism of thyroid control of drug metabolism is unclear but may involve changes in cytochrome P450, although not all changes in enzyme activity

Table 4.8 Sex dependency of the effect of thyroidectomy on hepatic drug metabolism

	Effect of thyroidectomy	
Enzyme activity	**Male animals**	**Female animals**
Alcohol oxidation	(Not determined)	Increase
Cytochrome P450	Increase	Increase
Ethylmorphine N-demethylase	Decrease	Decrease
Benzo[a]pyrene hydroxylase	Decrease	Decrease
Aniline 4-hydroxylase	Decrease	Decrease
5β-Reductase	(No change)	Increase
11β-Hydroxysteroid dehydrogenase	Decrease	Increase

(Data from various sources; see further reading section in Chapter 5.)

Animal	1-Naphthol glucuronide formed (min^{-1} g^{-1} liver)[a]
Control male	1.70 ± 0.17
TX male	1.27 ± 0.12*
Control female	0.59 ± 0.08
TX female	0.34 ± 0.03*

Table 4.9 The effect of thyroidectomy (TX) on glucuronidation of 1-naphthol in liver cubes

[a] Results expressed as mean ± (standard deviation)
* = $p < 0.05$.

are correlated with changes in cytochrome P450. Other changes that have been reported are an increase in haem oxygenase (which degrades cytochrome P450) and changes in inducibility in thyroidectomised animals, although the induction of drug-metabolising enzymes by TCDD does not seem to be related to the effect of TCDD on thyroid status. Changes in CYPs 2C11 and 3A2 in the rat induced by retinal are, however, related to the ability of this compound to alter thyroid status.

Phase 2 metabolism can also be affected by thyroidectomy – the glucuronidation of 1-naphthol is significantly lower in thyroidectomised rats of both sexes (Table 4.9). Sulfotransferase activities are also thyroid-dependent.

Thus the thyroid glands may play a role in the hormonal control of drug metabolism and, in the rat, may be involved in the sexual differentiation of drug metabolism.

4.5.6 Pancreas

The pancreas produces and secretes one hormone of particular relevance to the control of drug metabolism, i.e. insulin. This is produced by the β-cells of the endocrine pancreas.

Diabetes mellitus (a reduction in the amount or action of insulin caused by genetic abnormalities or chemically by means of streptozotocin) causes marked changes in hepatic phase 1 and 2 metabolism (see Table 4.10).

Phase 1 metabolism in the liver, exemplified by diazepam and lignocaine hydroxylation and N-dealkylation, shows a marked decrease in activity (except lidocaine 3-hydroxylation) in diabetic rats whereas enzyme activities in the intestine rise. As usual in the rat, the sex of the animal must be taken into consideration – all of the effects noted are only seen in the male. Replacement therapy with insulin can reverse the effects of diabetes caused by streptozotocin (see Figure 4.11). Studies using isolated hepatocytes have confirmed that the effect of insulin is direct on the liver in some cases and in others the effect is secondary to the metabolic changes induced by diabetes (i.e. ketone production inducing CYP2E1) or other hormonal changes (such as alteration of GH secretion – the effects of which are noted above). The diabetes-inducible cytochrome P450 is recognised to be CYP2E1, which is also induced by acetone. The expression of the CYP2C12 gene, however, can be decreased by insulin through interaction with specific insulin response elements.

Table 4.10 The effect of streptozotocin (STZ)-induced diabetes on liver weight, blood glucose and drug metabolism in the male rat

	Control	STZ-treated	
Liver (% body weight)	3.58 ± 0.28^a	4.32 ± 0.47	**
Blood glucose (mM)	8.67 ± 0.68	32.13 ± 2.54	***
Cytochrome P450 (nmoles mg^{-1})	0.56 ± 0.06	0.54 ± 0.08	n.s.
Diazepam 3-hydroxylase (pmoles min^{-1} g^{-1} protein)	60.3 ± 21.4	35.6 ± 4.8	*
Diazepam N-demethylase (pmoles min^{-1} g^{-1} protein)	32.4 ± 7.6	19.4 ± 5.1	*
Lignocaine 3-hydroxylase (pmoles min^{-1} g^{-1} protein)	35 ± 6	31 ± 16	n.s.
Lignocaine N-de-ethylase (pmoles min^{-1} g^{-1} protein)	317 ± 118	182 ± 65	*
1-Naphthol glucuronidation (nmoles product min^{-1} g^{-1} liver)	1.42 ± 0.22	1.57 ± 0.15	n.s.

^{a} Mean $\pm$ S.D. (of at least 4 values)
* $= p < 0.05$; ** $= p < 0.01$; *** $= p < 0.001$; n.s. $=$ not significant, $p > 0.05$.

It would appear that thyroid, pituitary and adrenal hormones (except adrenal androgens), estrogens and insulin can act directly on the liver, whereas androgens exert their effects on the liver by interaction with the hypothalamo-hypophyseal axis, modifying the release of pituitary hormones.

The hormonal control of drug metabolism is, as can be seen from the above summary, quite complex and is made more so by the numerous interactions of the hormones involved (e.g. GH and insulin have been shown to be mutually

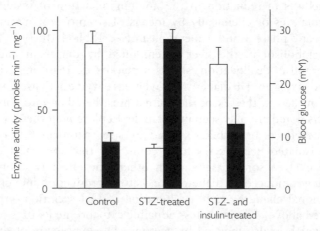

Figure 4.11 The effect of streptozotocin (STZ) and insulin treatment on blood glucose levels and the N-de-ethylation of lignocaine in the rat liver. Plain block diagrams represent enzyme activity; filled blocks, blood glucose.

Table 4.11 The effect of pregnancy on the metabolism of coumarin and progesterone in the rat

	Non-pregnant	Pregnant
Coumarin 3-hydroxylase	18.61 ± 1.92	10.28 ± 1.05*
Progesterone 16α-hydroxylase	6.68 ± 0.15	4.63 ± 0.33*
Progesterone 5α-reductase	15.38 ± 0.26	21.86 ± 0.47*

Results expressed as nmoles product $h^{-1} g^{-1}$ protein; mean ± (standard deviation)
* = $p < 0.05$
(From Kordish, R. and Feuer, G. (1972) *Biol. Neonate* **20**, 58–67, modified. Used with permission of S. Karger AG, Basel.)

antagonistic). No one hormone can be considered in isolation. Hormonal control is considered of major importance when examining drug metabolism in rodents and some farm species but is little considered in clinical practice.

4.5.7 Pregnancy

Pregnancy is a natural condition when the hormonal balance of the female body is grossly altered. The oestrous (menstrual) cycle ceases and there are large changes in blood levels of peptide and steroid hormones. It is relevant, therefore, to discuss the effects of pregnancy on drug metabolism under the heading of Hormonal Control.

In the rat, pregnancy causes a general decrease in drug metabolism, e.g. 3-hydroxylation of coumarin, but a more complex change in the metabolism of the endogenous progestagen, progesterone (Table 4.11).

These changes are thought to be due to progesterone or its metabolites that are found in blood in high concentrations during pregnancy. This is the same phenomenon seen in suckling infants (see Section 4.4) where progestagens in the mother's milk are thought to inhibit drug metabolism in the young animal in certain cases.

The study of drug metabolism during pregnancy in the human is more difficult due to the obvious ethical considerations of administering drugs to a pregnant woman. One study has shown, however, that CYP2D6 (discussed in Section 4.3 above) is induced in pregnancy, leading to a higher clearance of drugs such as metoprolol.

4.6 THE EFFECTS OF DISEASE ON DRUG METABOLISM

Many disease states have been shown to affect the way in which the body clears drugs and these are listed in Table 4.12. It can be seen that the major effects are observed with diseases affecting the liver. This is hardly surprising as the liver is quantitatively the most important site of drug biotransformation. Other diseases, however, such as infections and endocrine disorders, are also important when looking at drug metabolism.

Table 4.12 Disease states that affect drug metabolism

Cirrhosis of the liver
Alcoholic liver disease
Cholestatic jaundice
Liver carcinoma
Endocrine disorders
Diabetes mellitus
Hypo- and hyperthyroidism
Acromegaly
Pituitary dwarfism
Infections
Bacterial
Viral
Malaria
Inflammation

4.6.1 Cirrhosis

In cirrhosis parts of the liver are replaced by fibrous tissue and the number of functional hepatocytes is reduced. It is therefore not unexpected that drug metabolism is impaired in this condition and, indeed, the oxidative metabolism of chlordiazepoxide to its primary metabolite, desmethylchlordiazepoxide, is slower in cirrhotic patients.

This appears to be true also for the conversion of diazepam to desmethyldiazepam. Oxazepam and lorazepam metabolism, however, which is purely glucuronidation, is not affected by cirrhosis. The N-dealkylation of lignocaine is grossly affected by cirrhosis as is the oxidation of propranolol with a much longer half-life for each drug. The same increase in elimination half-life is seen for theophylline and tolbutamide (an oral hypoglycaemic). The problem of equating plasma half-life with metabolism is evident here as both lignocaine and propranolol are highly extracted drugs and, thus, the blood flow through the liver rather than the rate of metabolism is important (see Chapter 7).

Various drugs which are normally metabolised by the liver are not affected with respect to their metabolism by cirrhosis. Morphine, for example, is converted to its glucuronide by the liver and this conversion is unaffected by cirrhosis. In one instance the activation of a prodrug is impaired by cirrhosis. The conversion of prednisone (the prodrug) to prednisolone (the active drug) is slower in cirrhotic patients.

One other aspect of cirrhosis should also be considered and that is enzyme induction by drugs and other xenobiotics. It is well known that many drugs can increase the rate at which they and other drugs are metabolised (see Chapter 3). The cirrhotic condition can greatly diminish the degree of increase in drug metabolism. For example, phenobarbitone pretreatment of normal subjects markedly increases the metabolism of many drugs whereas similar pretreatment of cirrhotic patients has little effect.

Table 4.13 summarises the effect of cirrhosis on drug metabolism. It is noted that cirrhosis appears to depress phase 1 but has no effect on glucuronidation.

Table 4.13 The effect of liver cirrhosis on drug metabolism

Drugs affected	(Metabolic route)	Drugs not affected	(Metabolic route)
Chlordiazepoxide	(N-Demethylation)	Oxazepam	(Glucuronidation)
Diazepam	(N-Demethylation)	Lorazepam	(Glucuronidation)
Barbiturates	(Oxidation)	Morphine	(Glucuronidation)
Antipyrine	(Oxidation)	Paracetamol	(Glucuronidation)
Glutethimide	(Oxidation)		
Methadone	(Oxidation)		
Salicylates	(Glycine conjugation)		

(Data from various sources; see further reading section in Chapter 5.)

4.6.2 Alcoholic liver disease

Chronic alcohol administration can lead to a condition similar to that of cirrhosis with large portions of the liver replaced by fibrous masses following the death of the hepatocytes. Before this stage is reached, however, alcohol administration can markedly affect drug metabolism in different ways. The stages of alcohol's effects on drug metabolism are summarised in Figure 4.12.

Acute ethanol exposure ⟶ Chronic ethanol exposure ⟶ Alcoholic cirrhosis
(no hepatocellular changes)

Inhibition   Induction   Inhibition

Figure 4.12 The stages in the development of the effect of ethanol on hepatic drug metabolism.

Acute ethanol exposure in general decreases drug metabolism such that drugs metabolised primarily by phase 1 routes, e.g. chlordiazepoxide, diazepam, aminopyrine, pentobarbitone and chlorpromazine, or phase 2 routes, e.g. lorazepam, p-nitrophenol, harmol and paracetamol, exhibit longer half-lives if administered with ethanol. The inhibition of phase 1 metabolism is thought to be due to ethanol binding to cytochrome P450 (the liver actually has a cytochrome P450-dependent ethanol oxidising system (MEOS) – CYP2E1) in a competitive manner. Inhibition of electron flow from the reductase to cytochrome P450 has also been noted. The alteration of the $NADP^+/NADPH$ ratio and the disturbance of the lipid environment of the cells have also been put forward as possible explanations of the effects of ethanol on phase 1 metabolism.

The inhibition of phase 2 metabolism is not due to inhibition of the enzymes involved. In the case of glucuronidation, ethanol is thought to increase the $NADH/NAD^+$ ratio (via oxidation of ethanol by alcohol dehydrogenase). This in turn inhibits the production of the co-factor for glucuronidation, UDP-glucuronic acid (which requires NAD^+) (Figure 4.13).

In one reaction, acute ethanol administration has been shown to increase activity and that is the acetylation of sulfadimidine. No explanation for this effect has been given.

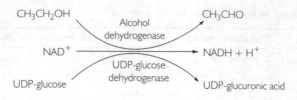

Figure 4.13 The interaction of ethanol with UDPGA production.

Chronic ethanol exposure in the absence of pathological change in the liver is usually associated with enhanced drug metabolism. Ethanol is classed as a microsomal enzyme inducer of a type different to both phenobarbitone and the polycyclic hydrocarbons (see Chapter 3). It has been shown to induce phase 1 and 2 metabolism. In terms of induction of cytochrome P450, ethanol is thought to cause an increase in the amount of CYP2E1 (the form also induced by acetone and in diabetes) and this leads to the marked increase in aniline 4-hydroxylase seen after ethanol exposure (Figure 4.14).

Once alcoholic liver disease has become extensive, a pattern of effects similar to cirrhosis is seen such that metabolism of diazepam, paracetamol and lignocaine is reduced.

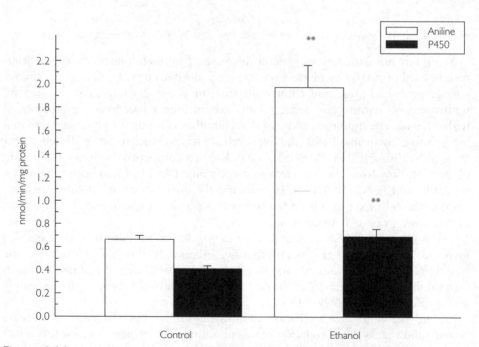

Figure 4.14 The effect of induction by ethanol inhalation on aniline 4-hydroxylase activity and total cytochrome P450 concentration in liver of rabbits.

4.6.3 Viral hepatitis

Little is known of the effects of viral hepatitis but what information is available suggests that this condition causes a decrease in hepatic drug metabolism. Chlordiazepoxide clearance is decreased in viral hepatitis, as is the clearance of meperidine (pethidine). Clearance of lignocaine is unaffected by viral hepatitis whereas tolbutamide exhibits an enhanced clearance in this condition. One study of patients with hepatitis A showed a marked decrease in the activity of CYP2A6 (related to 7-hydroxylation of coumarin).

4.6.4 Hepatoma

A hepatoma is a cancerous growth derived from the liver parenchymal cells. The drug-metabolising capacity of the tumour cells, however, is very much less than the corresponding normal cells. This is a typical loss of differentiated function in de-differentiated cells.

The loss of differentiated function is noted for the metabolism of aniline to 4-aminophenol. The level of aniline metabolism in the tumours was similar to that in foetal and regenerating liver.

The faster growing (i.e. less differentiated) the tumour the less drug metabolism was evident. This was shown particularly well with the 5α-reduction of testosterone (Table 4.14).

Metabolism of estrogens, methadone, benzphetamine and 4-nitroanisole are also found at much reduced levels in hepatoma tissue.

One interesting point emerged from these studies and that was that the unaffected liver tissue of the animal with the hepatoma also showed a reduced capacity to metabolise drugs. The decreases were not as dramatic as those of the hepatoma itself but the presence of a de-differentiated hepatoma could reduce hepatic drug metabolism by 20%. This has been challenged by Sultatos and Vessell who showed enhanced drug metabolism in liver tissue surrounding a hepatoma. The answer to this paradox lies, say the authors, in the fact that previous studies have used intramuscularly implanted hepatomas whereas they used intrahepatic hepatomas. This enhancement of drug metabolism in tumour-adjacent tissue would seem to extend to man (Table 4.15).

Table 4.14 The steroid 5α-reductase activity of various rat hepatomas

Hepatoma (code no.)		5α-Reductase activity (% vs control liver)
44		3.6
38B		2.6
7795	Growth rate increasing	2.0
5123A		1.5
7288C		1.0
7777		0.6
42A		0.2

(From Houglum, J.E. *et al.* (1974) *Cancer Res.* **34**, 938–941. Used with permission of the authors.

Table 4.15 Drug metabolism in hepatoma tissue and surrounding normal liver tissue

Tissue studied	Ethylmorphine N-demethylase (% vs control tissue)	Aniline hydroxylase (% vs control tissue)
Normal liver	100	100
Tumour	70	27
Tumour-adjacent liver	250	290
Far-removed liver	100	100

(From Sultatos, L.G. and Vessell, E.S. (1980) *P.N.A.S.* **77**, 600–603. Used with the permission of the authors.)

The changes in drug-metabolising capacity seen in hepatoma lines and liver adjacent to hepatomas are related to changes in cytochrome P450 levels – markedly decreased in hepatoma tissue but elevated in histologically normal liver tissue close to a tumour. Little difference appears to exist between the drug metabolising system of the tumour and normal tissue: each can be induced and inhibited similarly and, thus, the only difference lies in the amount of enzyme present.

4.6.5 Summary of effects of liver diseases on drug metabolism

As has been seen, diseases of various types generally decrease the liver's ability to metabolise drugs (with the notable exception of chronic ethanol exposure). The possible reasons for this decreased capacity are listed below:

1 decreased enzyme activity in liver
2 altered hepatic blood flow (intra/extrahepatic shunting)
3 hypoalbuminaemia (leading to lower plasma binding of drugs).

Of these reasons only (1) is really to be classed as a change in metabolism of the drug but the other two can lead to apparent changes in metabolism and, thus, must be considered.

Two theories have been put forward to explain the poor metabolism in cirrhotic patients: the 'sick cell' theory maintains that blood flow through the liver is normal but the cells are deficient in drug-metabolising enzymes, whereas the second theory, the 'intact hepatocyte' theory, says that the cells are normal but do not receive the normal blood flow due to shunting of blood past some parts of the liver (to get round the fibrous masses). Both theories have some evidence in favour of them, such as reduced cytochrome P450 levels and drug metabolising enzyme activity in cirrhotic rats ('sick cell' theory) and increased intrahepatic shunting (nine times normal) in cirrhotic animals ('intact hepatocyte' theory), and it is probable that both theories are correct and vary in importance, depending on the stage of cirrhosis and substrate, animal, etc., being studied.

4.6.6 Non-hepatic diseases

Other non-hepatic diseases should also be considered in terms of their influence on drug metabolism and these particularly include the hormonal diseases such as hyperthyroidism, pituitary insufficiency (dwarfism), adrenal insufficiency, pituitary, thyroid or adrenal tumours, diabetes, and the genetic abnormalities of sexual development. All of the above-mentioned disease states have been shown to influence drug metabolism (most of which have been discussed to a greater or lesser extent in Section 4.5).

More recently it has become obvious that general infectious diseases can affect drug metabolism. For instance, *Listeria monocytogenes* infection can dramatically reduce aminopyrine N-demethylase activity (to less than 10% of control) within 2 days and this is accompanied by a similar drop in cytochrome P450 content. Haem oxygenase activity rises during this period, perhaps indicating that cytochrome P450 degradation is to blame for the fall in enzyme content. A similar effect is seen with malarial or viral infections, inflammation and with treatment with endotoxin. The common feature in all cases is an activation of the host defence mechanisms in the body. It is now clear that cytokines are the common link in the effect of all of these conditions on drug metabolism.

Extensive work by Morgan has shown a central role of interferons in the control of cytochrome P450-related oxidative drug metabolism. The control is complex, involving many different cytokines as well as interactions between the different cell types in the liver (primarily hepatocytes and Kuppfer cells). The effects are dependent on the form of cytochrome P450 investigated. The signalling pathways appear to involve nitric oxide, peroxisome-proliferator activated receptors, interleukins and eicosanoids. Some effects, however, seem to be nitric oxide independent, such as the down-regulation of expression of the CYP2C11 gene in rat hepatocytes by interleukin-1β and endotoxin.

Endotoxin treatment has also been shown to depress expression of cytochrome P450 in women with the clearance of probe substrates, antipyrine (a general probe for cytochromes P450), hexobarbital (CYP2C) and theophylline (CYP1A2), all markedly lower. The changes were correlated with rises in TNF-α and IL-6 in plasma of the patients.

The health of the individual can thus play a major role in the drug-metabolising capacity of the liver of that individual and, together with age, probably represents the major consideration when deciding the dose of drug to be given to a patient or, indeed, whether a drug should be given at all.

This chapter has shown how the physiological and pathological make-up of the animal can influence the way in which it metabolises drugs. In the next chapter we intend to discuss the other major controlling influences on drug metabolism: the external factors. Further reading for this chapter will be found at the end of Chapter 5.

5 FACTORS AFFECTING DRUG METABOLISM: EXTERNAL FACTORS

LEARNING OBJECTIVES

At the end of this chapter, you should be able to:

- Discuss, using examples and giving mechanisms, how dietary nutritional factors (protein, fat, carbohydrate, minerals and vitamins) may affect drug metabolism
- Discuss, using examples and giving mechanisms, how dietary non-nutrients may affect drug metabolism
- Discuss, using examples and giving mechanisms, how environmental factors (heavy metals, industrial pollutants, pesticides and motor cycle exhaust) may affect drug metabolism
- Assess how the above factors may affect the intensity, duration of action and toxicity of drugs by affecting their metabolism

In the previous chapter, the physiological and pathological factors affecting drug metabolism were discussed. There are, however, other factors, from outside the body, that can also have a profound influence on drug metabolism. The body can be exposed to these factors by design (e.g. substances taken as food, alcohol and tobacco smoke) or by accident (air, water and food contaminants or pollutants). The first group will be referred to as dietary factors and the second group as environmental factors. The types of substances under each heading are listed in Table 5.1.

5.1 DIETARY FACTORS

In discussing dietary factors, two major groups of substances can be distinguished: the macronutrients (e.g. protein, carbohydrate and fats, making up the bulk of

Table 5.1 External factors affecting drug metabolism

Dietary factors	Environmental factors
Protein	Petroleum products
Fat	Pyrolysis products
Carbohydrate	Heavy metals
Vitamins	Insecticides, herbicides
Trace elements	Industrial pollutants
Pyrolysis products	Motor vehicle exhaust
Tobacco smoke	
Alcohol	

the diet) and micronutrients (vitamins and minerals, essential in small quantities). Dietary factors can also be said to include alcohol (which provides a large number of calories and is discussed in Section 4.6), non-nutrients (such as colourants, antioxidants and flavour components) and the components of tobacco smoke. Although the latter is not strictly a dietary factor, it is taken intentionally and has similar effects to some of the other non-nutrients in the diet.

5.1.1 Macronutrients

5.1.1.1 Protein

The normal proportion of protein in the diet is about 20% – animals kept on a diet containing this amount of protein show normal development of drug-metabolising enzymes. If, however, rats are fed on a 5% protein (casein) diet then oxidative drug-metabolising capacity decreases (Table 5.2). The decrease in drug metabolism is partially due to decreases in overall microsomal protein and partially to specific effects on the enzymes still remaining. Work by Campbell *et al.*, using isolated mixed-function oxidase components (cytochrome P450, reductase and phospholipid) in crossover experiments, has indicated that it is an alteration in the cytochrome P450 and not the reductase or lipid component that is responsible for the decrease in drug metabolism. It was suggested that the interaction of the cytochrome P450 with the reductase was affected in protein restriction.

This is confirmed by more recent data examining the changes in cytochrome P450 complement in severe protein deficiency in rats. Using Western blotting techniques, the level of CYP3A was seen to fall dramatically on reducing protein intake from 18% to 1%, whereas CYP1A2 only fell with a 0.5% protein diet and CYP1A1 did not show any fall. The changes in cytochrome P450 forms correlated well with changes in the metabolism of probe substrates such as progesterone. The flavin-dependent enzymes (e.g. 17-oxosteroid oxidoreductase) were not affected by protein malnutrition.

A similar effect of protein restriction is seen in man with decreases in aminopyrine and theophylline metabolism. For theophylline clearance a decrease of about 30% is seen when changing from a 20% to a 10% protein diet.

The effect of protein deficiency on phase 2 drug metabolism is more complex, with some activities decreasing, e.g. paracetamol (acetaminophen) glucuronidation, while others increase, e.g. 4-nitrophenol glucuronidation. For glutahione-*S*-transferase an alteration in subunit composition is seen when a protein-depletion diet is used.

	Enzyme activity (nmoles HCHO per 100 g bw per 10 min)
Control (20% casein)	10.5
5% Casein (4 days)	6.0
5% Casein (8 days)	<1.0

Table 5.2 The effect of feeding a 5% and 20% casein diet on the hepatic ethylmorphine N-demethylase activity in the rat

5.1.1.2 Fat

Lipids are required by the drug-metabolising enzymes as membrane components and, possibly, for specific interactions and certain lipid components can also act as inhibitors of drug metabolism (e.g. steroids, discussed in Chapter 4). How would a fat-deficient diet, therefore, affect drug metabolism?

It is seen that diets deficient in the essential fatty acids, notably linoleic acid, cause a reduction in the metabolism of ethylmorphine and hexobarbitone in the liver, and that subsequent addition of corn oil (containing linoleic acid) to the diet could reverse this effect. It is linoleic acid and arachidonic acid that seem to be particularly important in the control of drug metabolism. Treatment with corn oil or polyunsaturated fatty acids, for instance, increases microsomal content of these fatty acids and also increases drug-metabolising capacity, whereas replacement with saturated fats (e.g. stearic acid or beef tallow) does not have this effect. The effects may be different for different tissues – for example, a high-fat diet can decrease arylhydrocarbon hydroxylase in the lung while increasing the same activity in the kidney and having no effect in the liver.

Various explanations of these effects have been put forward, such as the theory that essential fatty acids are needed for the interaction of substrate with the active site of cytochrome P450, the essential fatty acids in this case being incorporated into phospholipids. No consistent effects of deprivation of, or supplementation with, essential fatty acids on substrate binding to cytochrome P450 have been seen. An effect mediated via a direct effect on the amount of cytochrome P450 has also been postulated, as deficiencies in essential fatty acids lead to decreased concentrations of cytochrome P450 in some instances (see Figure 5.1).

Feeding rats cholesterol, a major component of the endoplasmic reticulum membrane, reduces the overall concentration of cytochrome P450 in the membrane, which correlates with a fall in aminopyrine N-demethylase activity.

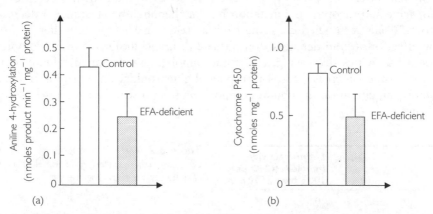

Figure 5.1 The effect of essential fatty acid (EFA) deficiency on (a) aniline 4-hydroxylation and (b) cytochrome P450 levels in liver. (From Kaschnitz, R. (1970) *Hoppe-Seyler's Z. Physiol Chem.* **351**, 771–774. Used with permission of the author.

5.1.1.3 Carbohydrate

Carbohydrates seem to have few effects on drug metabolism, although a high intake of glucose in particular can inhibit barbiturate metabolism, and thus lengthen sleeping time. Glucose excess has also been shown to decrease hepatic cytochrome P450 content and to lower biphenyl-4-hydroxylase activity. It has been suggested that carbohydrate manipulations are effective by more diverse effects on intermediary metabolism and hormone balance, and not by a direct effect on the liver.

Although examples have been given of the effects of protein, fat and carbo-hydrate on drug metabolism, it is clear from the literature that the individual influences of these macronutrients is difficult to assess, as each affects the use of the other and, thus, an effect on one component may be due to changes it caused in another. Indeed, if isocaloric replacement is used then a high fat/low carbo-hydrate diet will be replaced by a low fat/high carbohydrate diet (to maintain the same number of calories) and, thus, the effect seen could be due to either change.

5.1.1.4 Starvation and re-feeding

This may be further illustrated by looking at one particular aspect of diet, starvation. Starvation of female rats causes marked rises in some enzyme activities (contrast this with the effect of isocaloric protein deficiency) while having little effect on other activities (Table 5.3) while in male rats there is a marked reduc-tion in aminopyrine N-demethylation and an increase in aniline 4-hydroxylation. It would appear that starvation can actually induce the synthesis of some micro-somal proteins in contrast to the marked loss of protein from the liver as a whole. The effects of starvation in the male rat can be directly related to the change in the cytochrome P450 profile – CYP2C11 falls (thus the decrease in aminopyrine metabolism) and CYP2E1 rises (thus the increase in aniline metabolism). The rise in CYP2E1 is most likely a result of the breakdown of fatty tissue releasing free fatty acids that are partially converted to ketone bodies (e.g. acetone) that are known to induce this enzyme (see the effect of diabetes in Chapter 4). It is interesting to note that over-feeding of rats (a good model of human obesity) also causes an increase in CYP2E1 for the same reason, i.e. excess free fatty acids in the blood (Figure 5.2).

In humans the effects of starvation and re-feeding are also somewhat confusing, with the clearance of paracetamol (acetaminophen), chloroquine and metranida-zole all decreased whereas in malnourished children, aspirin clearance may be enhanced.

Table 5.3 The effect of starvation on drug metabolism in rats

Enzyme	Change (%) after starvation
Aminopyrine N-demethylase	+114
4-Nitroanisole O-demethylase	+90
Aniline 4-hydroxylation	+94
Zoxazolamine hydroxylation	+15
Dichlorophenolindophenol reductase	+7

(Data from various sources: see further reading section at the end of this chapter.)

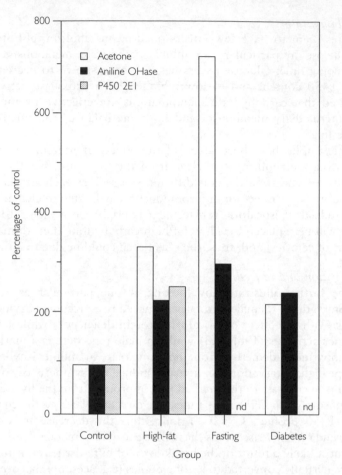

Figure 5.2 Effect of high-fat, fasting and diabetes mellitus on plasma acetone levels, hepatic aniline 4-hydroxylase activity and hepatic mRNA for cytochrome P450 2E1 in rats. nd = not determined. Data taken from Yun, Y-P. *et al.* (1992) *Mol. Pharmacol.*, **41**, 474–479.

It is therefore clear that changes in macronutrients can markedly affect the drug-metabolising capacity of the liver and other tissues but the effects are not always easily predicted.

Apart from the macronutrients noted above there are many other components of the diet that can affect drug metabolism. The most noticeable of these are the micronutrients: the vitamins and minerals and some of the non-nutrients found in food and drink.

5.1.2 Vitamins

Vitamins are an essential part of the diet and are needed for the synthesis of proteins and lipids, both of which are vital components of the drug metabolising

Vitamin A	***Table 5.4*** Vitamins affecting
Vitamin B group	drug metabolism
Thiamine (B$_1$)	
Riboflavin (B$_2$)	
Vitamin C	
Vitamin E	
Vitamin K	

enzyme system. It is therefore not surprising that changes in vitamin levels, particularly deficiencies, cause changes in drug-metabolising capacity. The vitamins indicated to be involved in drug metabolism are listed in Table 5.4.

5.1.2.1 Vitamin A

Retinoids (vitamin A and its metabolites) have been found to have profound effects on drug metabolism. The effects of the retinoids depend on whether they bind to the retinoic acid (RAR) or retinoid X (RXR) receptors. Ligands at the RXR receptor (e.g. the synthetic retinoid, Targretin) had a marked stimulatory effect on CYPs 2B1/2, 2C11, 3A and 4A whereas ligands at the RAR receptor (such as the naturally occurring Tretinoin) significantly decreased CYP1A2 and 3A whilst giving a smaller increase in CYP2C11 and 4A than the corresponding RXR-specific ligand (Figure 5.3). CYP2C7 is also induced by retinoids binding to the RAR receptor whereas down-regulation of CYP2C11 by vitamin A deficiency can be overcome by treatment with androgens. Vitamin A deficiency is also seen to cause a fall in circulating androgen levels but androgen treatment has no effect on circulating vitamin A levels.

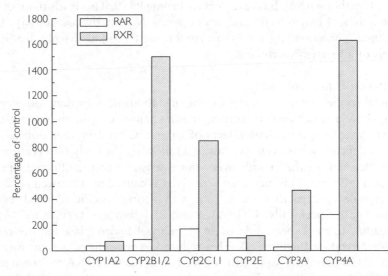

Figure 5.3 The effect of treatment with an RAR- or RXR-specific ligand on cytochrome P450 levels in rat liver.

In Syrian hamsters, vitamin A deficiency causes a fall in CYP2A1 and a concomitant decrease in testosterone 7α-hydroxylase activity. Supplementation with vitamin A (retinyl palmitate) restores the protein and enzyme activity to control levels.

5.1.2.2 Thiamine (vitamin B_1)

Thiamine deficiency has been shown to increase the metabolism of aniline and reduce hexobarbitone metabolism whereas excess thiamine inhibits aniline and ethylmorphine metabolism. The effect of thiamine is related to changes in the microsomal cytochromes (P450 and b_5) and NADPH-cytochrome P450 reductase levels. The effects were not similar to starvation although it was suggested that the effects of thiamine were mediated via a reduction in blood glucose. More recently thiamine has been found to change the type of cytochrome P450 present – an increase in CYP2E1 and reduction in CYP2C11 – and this could account for the effects seen.

5.1.2.3 Riboflavin (vitamin B_2)

A derivative of riboflavin is an essential component in the flavoprotein, NADPH-cytochrome P450 reductase, which is itself a component of the mixed-function oxidase system. A deficiency of riboflavin, therefore, would be expected to reduce NADPH-cytochrome P450 reductase content and thus decrease drug-metabolising capacity. This is seen for azo reduction of 4-dimethylaminoazobenzene in vitamin B_2-deficient rats, whereas aminopyrine N-demethylase shows an increase.

The degree of riboflavin deficiency may, however, complicate the interpretation of the data. Opposite effects of mild, short-term and severe, long-term deficiency of this vitamin on drug metabolism have been reported. Soon after the start of a riboflavin-deficient diet, a marked decrease in NADPH-cytochrome P450 reductase is seen, together with an increase in cytochrome P450. This leads to an overall increase in aniline 4-hydroxylase and aminopyrine N-demethylase activity. Later in the treatment, however, the levels of cytochrome P450 fall sharply, leading to lower levels of all enzyme activities.

5.1.2.4 Vitamin C (ascorbic acid)

Of the animal species studied in terms of drug metabolism, only man, monkey and guinea pig show a nutritional requirement for vitamin C and, thus, only these animals may be expected to show effects of vitamin C on drug metabolism.

Vitamin C deficiency has been well studied following the early observation that guinea pigs deficient in the vitamin were more sensitive to the effects of pentobarbitone and procaine. This increased sensitivity is caused by a marked reduction in drug-metabolising capacity concomitant with a form-specific reduced level of cytochrome P450. Specifically, CYP1A1/2 and 2E1 (but not CYP2B or 3A) are reduced, leading to the expected decrease in aniline 4-hydroxylase but not testosterone 6β-hydroxylase (Figure 5.4). This reduced expression of certain forms of cytochrome P450 correlates well with reduced amounts of mRNA for these forms in vitamin C-deficient animals. There is evidence to suggest that the deficiency of vitamin C may interfere with haem biosynthesis and, thus, affect cytochrome P450

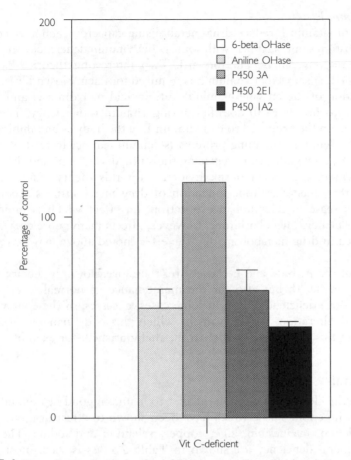

Vit C-deficient

Figure 5.4 The effects of vitamin C deficiency on aniline 4-hydroxylase and testosterone 6-hydroxylase activity and specific forms of cytochrome P450 in the guinea pig. Data taken from Kanazana, Y. et al. (1991) *Mol. Pharmacol.* **39**, 456–460.

levels. Abnormal binding spectra have also been seen in vitamin C-deficient guinea pigs – the binding spectra could be returned to normal using ascorbyl palmitate (the fatty acid derivative of vitamin C). It may, thus, be that vitamin C is involved in the maintenance of the membrane structure of the endoplasmic reticulum.

Ascorbic acid has also been reported to alleviate some of the changes in cytochrome P450 (notably the increase in CYP2E1) noted in diabetic rats. This is thought to be an action of vitamin C as an anti-oxidant, reducing the circulating levels of acetone, which is the likely cause of induction of CYP2E1 in diabetes (see Chapter 4).

In man, excess vitamin C ingestion decreases the ability of the gut to conjugate estrogens with sulfate. This is thought to be due to a competition of ascorbic acid and the estrogens for the limited supply of the cofactor required for sulfation (PAPS).

5.1.2.5 Vitamin E

Deficiencies of vitamin E reduce drug-metabolising capacity when assayed with a variety of substrates but, again, as with some other vitamin deficiencies, no definite biochemical reasons can be put forward. Two interesting theories have been advanced. The first states that vitamin E is required for haem biosynthesis, notably for the function of the enzyme δ-aminolevulinic acid dehydratase, and, indeed, microsomal cytochrome P450 does fall during vitamin E deficiency. The second theory is based on the proposed role of vitamin E in the body as an inhibitor of the oxidation of selenium-containing proteins (selenium can act instead of sulfur in some instances, a selenide group replacing the sulfhydryl group) and the need for such a protein in drug metabolism. Evidence for this theory comes from the observation that phenobarbitone induction of drug metabolism is accompanied by a large increase in selenium incorporation, an effect which is inhibited by vitamin E deficiency. Phenobarbitone, however, affects many more enzymes than those involved in drug metabolism, and the effect noted above may be related to one of those.

Vitamins of the A, B, C and E classes are, therefore, not only dietary requirements for good health but also for the maintenance of normal levels of drug metabolism. Both deficiencies and, in some cases, excesses, of these vitamins can cause marked alterations in the way in which the body handles drugs. The significance of this to clinical practice in the malnourished, for example, is clear.

5.1.3 Minerals

Minerals are the elements needed in the diet to maintain good health and normal physiological function. Those which have been shown to affect drug metabolism are iron, calcium, magnesium, zinc, copper, selenium and iodine. The overall effects of mineral deficiency are shown in Table 5.5. As is seen, most mineral deficiencies lead to a fall in drug metabolism.

Iron deficiency is an exception to the general rule, in that it causes an increase in drug-metabolising capacity (see Table 5.5). Excess iron in the diet can also inhibit drug metabolism. This is an unusual finding considering that iron is an essential component of the haem moiety of cytochrome P450 and, thus, would be expected to be essential for cytochrome P450 synthesis. Cytochrome P450 levels are, however, unchanged in iron deficiency. Iron levels in liver are inversely correlated to NADPH-dependent lipid peroxidation. As increased lipid peroxidation has been associated with decreased drug metabolism, this may offer an explanation of the effects of iron. Iron deficiency limits the degree of lipid peroxidation and thus allows more expression of the drug-metabolising enzymes. The active form of iron may be ferritin as ferritin added directly to microsomal incubations can inhibit aminopyrine and aniline metabolism. Iron-deficient diets markedly decrease intestinal drug metabolism, and this may be of greater pharmacological and toxicological importance considering the protective role of the intestinal enzymes, particularly against the procarcinogenic polycyclic hydrocarbons. This latter effect is associated with a fall in the levels of cytochrome P450 in this tissue.

Table 5.5 The effects of mineral deficiencies on hepatic drug metabolism

Mineral	Effect of deficiency on drug metabolism	Enzymes affected
Calcium	Decrease	Aminopyrine N-demethylase
	Decrease	Nitroreductase
	Decrease	Hexobarbitone oxidation
Magnesium	Decrease	Aniline 4-hydroxylation
	Decrease	Aminopyrine N-demethylase
	No change	Nitroreductase
	No change	Pentobarbitone oxidation
	Decrease	Cytochrome P450
Iron	Increase	Hexobarbitone oxidation
	Increase	Aminopyrine N-demethylation
	Increase	Cytochrome b_5
	No change	Cytochrome P450
	Increase/no change	Aniline 4-hydroxylation
	No change	Nitroreductase
	No change	Glucuronosyltransferase
Potassium	No change	Aniline 4-hydroxylation
	No change	Aminopyrine N-demethylation
	No change	Nitroreductase
Copper	Decrease	Aniline 4-hydroxylation
	Increase	Benzo[a]pyrene hydroxylation
	Decrease	Hexobarbitone oxidation
	Decrease	Zoxazolamine 6-hydroxylation
Zinc	Decrease	Aminopyrine N-demethylase
	Decrease	Pentobarbitone oxidation
	Decrease	Cytochrome P450
Selenium	No change	Ethylmorphine N-demethylase
	No change	Biphenyl 4-hydroxylase
	No change	Pentobarbitone oxidation
Iodine	Increase	Aminopyrine N-demethylase
	Increase	Hexobarbitone oxidation
	Increase	Benzo[a]pyrene hydroxylation
	Increase	Aniline 4-hydroxylation
	No change	Glucuronosyltransferase

(Data from various sources; see further reading section at the end of this chapter.)

Calcium and magnesium deficiency are associated with a decrease in drug metabolism, particularly phase 1 cytochrome P450-dependent metabolism such as aniline 4-hydroxylation and aminopyrine N-demethylation and, in the case of magnesium, drug glucuronidation. The effects of calcium deficiency take longer to develop than those of magnesium deficiency (40 days as opposed to 10 days). Magnesium deficiency, often found in conjunction with calcium deficiency, gives a specific effect and is not related to decreased food intake or starvation effects. Various explanations for the effect of magnesium deficiency have been put forward. Decreases in NADPH-cytochrome P450 reductase have been correlated to a reduced ability to metabolise drugs and decreased liver magnesium levels. In many studies, however, no decrease in liver magnesium levels is evident and alternative explanations are needed. One such explanation is found in the interaction of magnesium, thyroid hormones and phospholipids. Thyroid hormone levels are depressed in magnesium-depleted animals, a change that can lead to decreased drug metabolism (see Chapter 4). Magnesium-depleted diets also markedly reduce the microsomal content of lysophosphatidylcholine and, to a lesser extent, phosphatidylcholine – an effect also associated with decreased drug-metabolising capacity. The possibility that magnesium affects drug metabolism via thyroid hormones that act through an effect on phospholipid metabolism must be considered.

The effects of copper deficiency on drug metabolism are variable (see Table 5.5) and no consensus is evident on the mechanism of these effects. Alterations in NADPH-cytochrome P450 reductase or binding of substrate to cytochrome P450 have been put forward as possible mechanisms, but these do not explain all of the effects seen. One interesting effect of copper deficiency on drug metabolism is the toxicity of parathion. Parathion is normally metabolised to the toxic compound paraoxon or to the relatively non-toxic 4-nitrophenol. In copper-deficient mice, parathion is found to be more toxic than in normal mice due to a reduced ability to produce the non-toxic 4-nitrophenol, thus allowing more of the substance to be converted to paraoxon.

It is interesting to note that excess copper has the same effect as copper deficiency, i.e. a reduced ability to metabolise drugs in some cases. Thus an optimum level of dietary copper exists for the maintenance of drug metabolism in the body.

Zinc deficiency leads to reduced drug metabolism for some substrates (e.g. benzo[a]pyrene hydroxylation and aminopyrine N-demethylation) but no effects on others (e.g. aniline and zoxazolamine hydroxylation). The effects are related to reduced cytochrome P450 levels. There are also marked changes in phase 2 metabolism with falls in glutathione S-transferase and UDP-glucuronosyltransferase activities. Zinc-deficient diets lead to extreme poor health in animals and the effects seen may be a function of this malnutrition rather than a specific effect of zinc.

Excess zinc, however, has marked toxicological effects, giving significantly reduced hepatic cytochrome P450 levels.

Selenium, as an essential trace element, is linked to vitamin E and the effects of both on drug metabolism are closely related (see Section 5.1.2.5). Selenium deficiency impairs the ability of the liver to respond to phenobarbitone treatment. In the presence of selenium a 3.65-fold induction is seen but this falls to 2.64-fold in selenium-deficient animals. Selenium deficiency has also been shown to markedly inhibit expression of the estrogen sulfotransferase gene in the rat (to less than 10% of control).

It can thus be seen that a deficiency (or, to a lesser extent, an excess) of many micronutrients can have noticeable effects on drug metabolism. The whole subject of the interaction of dietary components and drug metabolism can become extremely complex as the effects of nutritional elements can overlap and involve other control mechanisms such as the hormones. A summary of the effects of macro- and micronutrients is given in Figure 5.5.

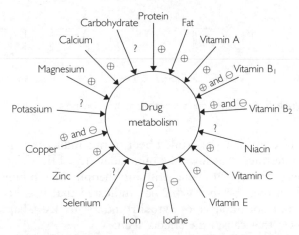

Figure 5.5 The effects of dietary nutrients on drug metabolism: a summary. Key: $\oplus$ = an increase in drug metabolism; $\ominus$ = a decrease in drug metabolism.

The importance of nutritional factors on drug metabolism is greatest in conditions of deficiency and, thus, in cases of malnutrition. As this is particularly prevalent in Third World societies, it is here that these effects are most often encountered but where funding is deficient to study and counteract the effects.

5.1.4 Non-nutrients

When dealing with the effects of diet on drug metabolism, it must be remembered that food contains not only nutritional factors (discussed above) but also other chemical substances, and any examination of diet-related effects on drug metabolism should include studies on these substances. The most notable group of these substances naturally occurring in food which affect drug metabolism are the pyrolysis products – chemicals formed by the cooking (literally burning) of the food.

The pyrolysis products that are formed in meat and fish, particularly when fried or charcoal-broiled, have been isolated as breakdown products of amino acids, mainly tryptophan. The structures of some of them are shown in Figure 5.6. All these compounds are known inducers of CYP1A1 (aryl hydrocarbon hydroxylase) and are also potential mutagens/carcinogens.

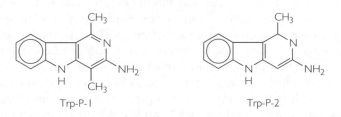

Figure 5.6 Tryptophan pyrolysis products found in fried or charcoal-broiled meat and fish.

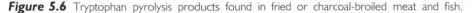

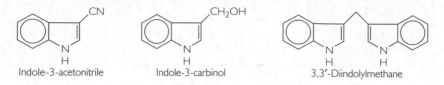

Figure 5.7 Indoles found in cabbage and Brussels sprouts.

It is found that feeding charcoal-broiled beef to rats induces the metabolism of phenacetin in the intestines, thus lowering bioavailability of the drug. A fall is also seen in plasma concentrations of phenacetin and theophylline in humans fed on a charcoal-broiled beef diet. Further work has indicated that it is benzo[a]pyrene (a polycyclic hydrocarbon inducer of cytochrome P450; see Chapter 3) in the charcoal-broiled beef that causes the effects seen.

One other group of compounds that could also be considered in this category are the substances found in cabbages and Brussels sprouts (Brassica). These compounds are of the indole type (Figure 5.7) and are also seen to be enzyme inducers. Their similarity to the tryptophan pyrolysis products is noticeable. Dietary Brussels sprouts and cabbage induce the hydroxylation of benzo[a]pyrene and hexobarbitone, the O-dealkylation of phenacetin (see above) and 7-ethoxycoumarin in the rat. Other vegetables not containing indoles do not induce drug metabolism. Studies in humans have shown a similar induction of caffeine metabolism following short-term dietary supplementation with Brassica vegetables. It has been suggested that the induction of CYP1A2 may be responsible for the alterations in metabolism seen. A similar increase in glucuronidation of paracetamol (acetaminophen) is also seen following ingestion of cabbage and Brussels sprouts.

A more recent and fascinating discovery is the marked effect of grapefruit juice (but not other citrus fruit juices) on drug metabolism. Grapefruit juice inhibits human CYPs 3A4, 1A2 and 2A6 *in vitro*, which would explain the reduced clearance of such drugs as cyclosporine, terfenadine and caffeine. The mechanism of this effect has been the subject of intense research, with many components of grapefruit juice being put forward as candidates for action. The flavanoids extracted from grapefruit juice (e.g. naringenin) were initially considered the active component as they could inhibit 6β-hydroxylation of testosterone (a probe for CYP3A4) in human liver microsomes. Flavanoids are well recognised as inhibitors of cytochrome P450 with many plant-derived flavanoids having form-specific effects. Other phytochemicals can also inhibit cytochrome P450 (e.g. curcumin from turmeric and diallyl sulfide from garlic). Evidence is building up, however, that grapefruit juice contains a suicide substrate for CYP3A4 (one candidate group of compounds are the furocoumarin dimers) which reduces the enzyme activity in the intestines, thus leading to enhanced bioavailability of numerous drugs.

Thus, even non-nutrient components of food can have marked effects on drug metabolism. It is likely that many more non-nutrient components of the diet (such as colourings, flavourings, food additives) can act as inducers or inhibitors of drug metabolism and that this is a common phenomenon.

5.1.5 Tobacco smoking

One other 'dietary' component can be considered: tobacco smoke. Although not strictly a food component, tobacco smoke is inhaled deliberately and, thus, is a self-inflicted effector of drug metabolism. Tobacco smoking can be thought of as a different way of ingesting pyrolysis products (from the burning of the plant materials in tobacco) with the lungs the first site of interaction rather than the intestine as in the case of charcoal-broiled meat. The most common effect of tobacco smoking is an increase in biotransformation of drugs – an effect very similar to that seen for ingestion of charcoal-broiled meat. Indeed, there is a common factor: the polycyclic hydrocarbon benzo[*a*]pyrene – this substance is found in both charcoal-broiled meat and tobacco smoke.

A marked effect on the plasma phenacetin level can be seen following tobacco smoking (cf. the effect of charcoal-broiled meat on phenacetin plasma levels) (Figure 5.8). The lower plasma level of phenacetin was due to increased metabolism either by the intestinal mucosa or 'first-pass' through the liver.

Another well-studied drug marker is antipyrine, the metabolism of which is directly related to its rate of excretion. Using antipyrine as a substrate, smoking was found to increase drug clearance and thus, by inference, the rate of metabolism of antipyrine. Stopping smoking returns the rate of metabolism of antipyrine to the pre-smoking level. The metabolism of a number of other probe drugs is affected by smoking, e.g. ethoxyresorufin (dealkylated by CYP1A), pentoxyresorufin (CYP2B), chlorzoxazone (CYP2E1) and erythromycin (CYP3A). Phase 2 metabolism has also been shown to be affected by tobacco smoking (see Table 5.6). Thus tobacco smoking selectively induces the metabolism of some drugs. Tobacco smoke contains at least 3000 different chemicals, some of which are known enzyme inducers (such as the polycyclic hydrocarbons discussed above) and some known enzyme

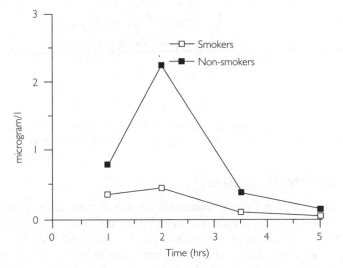

Figure 5.8 Mean plasma concentrations of phenacetin as a function of time in smokers and non-smokers. (Data from Pantuck, E.J. *et al.* (1972) *Science* **175**, 1248–1250.)

Table 5.6 The effect of tobacco smoking on the metabolism of drugs

Affected (increased)	Not affected
Nicotine	Diazepam
Theophylline	Phenytoin
Imipramine	Warfarin
Pentazocine	Nortriptyline

inhibitors (e.g. carbon monoxide, hydrogen cyanide). From the results obtained it is the inductive effects of tobacco smoke that are prevalent. Animal experiments have indicated that the great majority, if not all, of the effects of tobacco smoking can be mimicked by treatment with benzo[*a*]pyrene (see Chapter 3). It thus seems likely that the major effects of tobacco smoking are due to induction of drug metabolism by benzo[*a*]pyrene and other such compounds. Marijuana smoking produces identical effects to tobacco smoking and cannot be looked upon as a 'safer' habit in this respect.

A summary of the effects of the non-nutrient compounds of the diet on drug metabolism is given in Figure 5.9. It should be remembered that there are many more dietary non-nutrients such as colourants, anti-oxidants and flavourings which could also influence drug metabolism. Space limitations, however, restrict our coverage of this extensive subject.

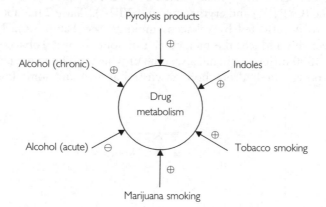

Figure 5.9 The influence of dietary non-nutrients on drug metabolism: a summary. Key: ⊕ = an increase in drug metabolism; ⊖ = a decrease in drug metabolism.

5.2 ENVIRONMENTAL FACTORS

Environmental factors are those influences in our surroundings that can affect drug metabolism; no conscious act is required to be influenced by them (cf. dietary factors) but the effects on drug metabolism can be profound. The environment is replete with substances that can affect drug metabolism and reviewers have different views concerning what constitutes an environmental factor. Many include dietary factors in this category and one should not be confused by these differences in nomenclature. It should also be realised that there are a large number of environmental chemicals that could potentially affect drug metabolism; the representative examples of a number of groups of compounds discussed here are only a small part of this. Those chemicals to be considered in this section are:

Heavy metals: lead, mercury, cadmium, gadolinium.
Industrial pollutants: tetrachlorodibenzodioxin (TCDD), solvents, polychlorinated biphenyls (PCBs).
Insecticides, herbicides: parathion, mirex.
Motor vehicle exhaust.

5.2.1 Heavy metals

Exposure of the human population to heavy metals can be related to occupation (cadmium from zinc smelting), diet (such as cadmium in vegetables) or other phenomena (e.g. lead in water from lead pipes). Most exposure is low level and long term and so cumulative exposure becomes important. These facts are rarely taken into account when examining heavy metal effects on drug metabolism in experimental animals.

Chronic exposure of rats to lead in the diet has little effect on drug metabolising capacity but does induce cytochrome P450 levels. The increased level of cytochrome P450 indicates that lead induces a form of enzyme that does not metabolise any of the substrates so far tested – different substrates may show induction of drug-metabolising capacity. Acute lead toxicity in rats, however, is associated with reduced drug-metabolising capacity. The situation found in human subjects was similar but only young children exhibited the inhibition of drug metabolism during acute lead toxicity. No measurement of cytochrome P450 in humans was performed; thus, the possible induction of this enzyme by chronic lead exposure is still open to investigation.

Two possible explanations for the effect of acute lead exposure on drug metabolism have been put forward. If lead is added to incubations of microsomes the activity of NADPH-cytochrome P450 reductase is inhibited and this could lead to inhibition of drug metabolism with certain substrates. Lead has also been shown to inhibit one of the enzymes involved in the synthesis of haem, γ-aminolevulinic acid dehydratase, and thus could inhibit the production of the haem moiety in cytochrome P450.

Little work has been done on mercury's effects on drug metabolism: what has been done has used excessively high doses of this toxic metal. Inorganic forms of mercury (Hg^{2+}) seem to induce drug metabolism whereas organic mercury (methylmercury) inhibits drug metabolism after chronic administration. No explanations for the effects of mercury were found.

The great majority of the work published on the interaction of heavy metals with drug metabolism has been done with cadmium. This is an industrial pollutant in the manufacture of a number of metals including zinc, and is a dietary pollutant in vegetables grown in cadmium-rich soil. High intake of cadmium has been shown to be associated with inhibition of drug-metabolising enzymes. In the rat,

Table 5.7 The effect of cadmium on hepatic drug metabolism in male and female rats

Enzyme	Change (%) in enzyme activities caused by cadmium	
	Male	Female
Diazepam 3-hydroxylase	−58	+65
Diazepam N-demethylase	−55	+66
Imipramine 2-hydroxylase	−33	+9
Imipramine N-demethylase	−55	−4
Imipramine N-oxidase	−60	+7
Cytochrome P450	−25	+3

however, an interesting sexual dimorphism of the effect has been seen (Table 5.7). The male rat responds to cadmium treatment with marked inhibition of all enzyme activities studied and a concomitant decrease in cytochrome P450 levels. The female rat, on the other hand, shows no reduction in cytochrome P450 levels and, indeed, marked induction of diazepam metabolism.

A hormonal control of cadmium sensitivity similar to that of drug metabolism in general (see Chapter 4) was found to operate, i.e. removal of androgens from the male by castration removed their sensitivity to cadmium.

Cadmium was shown to have many effects on the various components of the drug metabolising enzyme system. Cytochrome P450 and cytochrome b_5 levels were reduced, and cytochrome P450 could be converted to the inactive cytochrome P420 *in vitro*. The former effect seems to be due to cadmium's ability to induce haem oxygenase activity (the enzyme that breaks down the haem of cytochromes P450 and b_5). The fact that only males respond to cadmium with marked inhibition of drug metabolism suggests that the cadmium-sensitive cytochrome P450 (or b_5) is sex-related. The alternative explanation, that cadmium exerts its effects by reducing androgen levels, does not hold, as androgen replacement therapy cannot reverse the effects of cadmium although it is known that cadmium causes massive testicular damage and does drastically reduce plasma testosterone levels (Table 5.8).

So cadmium not only reduces plasma testosterone levels but also makes the liver non-responsive to androgens. Little work has been done on the inducing ability of cadmium in the female rat although it has been suggested that the female is less sensitive to the toxic effects of cadmium by virtue of having a cadmium-binding protein which takes up the metal and prevents it being toxic.

Gadolinium is an interesting rare earth metal ion (Gd^{3+}) in that it inhibits the activity of the Kupffer cells in the liver. Other lanthanides have been shown to decrease cytochrome P450 activity, although gadolinium was thought to exert its protective action against carbon tetrachloride-induced hepatotoxicity by reducing the secretion of cytokines (previously shown to inhibit certain forms of cytochrome P450 – see Chapter 4). Evidence exists, however, that gadolinium also decreases cytochrome P450 and metabolism of the probe substrate, aniline.

Table 5.8 The effect of cadmium and testosterone treatment on hepatic drug metabolism in the male rat

Parameter	+Cd (% vs control)	+Cd +testosterone (% vs control)
Cytochrome P450	82	71
Diazepam 3-hydroxylase	75	72
Diazepam N-demethylase	64	66
Lignocaine 3-hydroxylase	292	229
Lignocaine N-de-ethylase	69	53
Plasma testosterone	17	78

Heavy metals can, therefore, induce and/or inhibit drug metabolism depending on the species and sex of animal and substrate studied. The relevance of this animal data to the environmentally encountered low-level, long-term exposure is debatable and much more work is needed to ascertain the effects of environmental exposure to these metals.

5.2.2 Industrial pollutants

There are literally thousands of industrial pollutants that, in experimental animals, have been shown to affect drug metabolism; the toxicological literature is full of such examples (see Chapter 6). Three important and well-studied industrial pollutants will be discussed in detail to illustrate the general principles; these are 2,3,7,8-tetrachlorodibenzo-*p*-dioxin (TCDD), industrial solvents of the benzene and chlorinated hydrocarbon types, and polychlorinated biphenyls (PCBs).

5.2.2.1 TCDD

TCDD is a polycyclic compound (Figure 5.10) with a rigid planar structure. It is a precursor for a number of herbicides and was the toxin released in the Seveso incident in Italy, causing widespread chloracne and fears for the future welfare of the population exposed to the chemical.

TCDD causes marked induction of the metabolism of polycyclic hydrocarbons and of the enzymes UDP-glucuronosyltransferase, γ-aminolevulinic acid synthetase and glutathione-*S*-transferase; it can thus affect both phase 1 and 2 metabolism. The mechanism of action of TCDD in inducing aryl hydrocarbon hydroxylase has been particularly studied. TCDD has a specific receptor in the liver cytosol (a classical DNA-linked receptor similar to that for the steroid hormones). Once

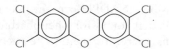

2,3,7,8-Tetrachlorodibenzo-*p*-dioxin (TCDD)

Figure 5.10 The structure of TCDD.

bound to the receptor, TCDD is taken to the nucleus where it interacts with DNA and, thus, gives its induction effects. This is very similar to the activation of the 'Ah locus' and is very probably the same system (see Chapter 3) leading to the induction of CYP1A1, amongst other effects.

5.2.2.2 Solvents

Solvents are in very widespread use in industry (and in the home). Serious concern is now being expressed about their effects on the body. The two groups of solvents of most interest in the study of drug metabolism are the benzene derivatives (benzene, toluene and the xylenes) and the chlorinated hydrocarbons (chloroform, trichloroethylene and dichloromethane).

The aromatic hydrocarbons (Figure 5.11) have been shown to induce cyto-chrome P450-dependent enzymes in the liver but have little effect on conjugation with glucuronic acid except after long-term exposure, when induction is also seen. As human exposure to these solvents is mainly by inhalation, experiments in animals tend to be inhalation experiments as well. Levels of solvent around the maximum allowed in industrial atmospheres are used so that an extrapolation of the data to man can be attempted; species differences have, however, to be taken into account here.

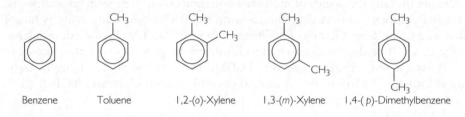

Benzene   Toluene   1,2-(o)-Xylene   1,3-(m)-Xylene   1,4-(p)-Dimethylbenzene

Figure 5.11 The structures of some aromatic hydrocarbons.

Xylene has also been shown to be an inducer of cytochrome P450 when administered by inhalation. Use of the individual components of the xylene mixture indicated that p-xylene (1,4-dimethylbenzene) was less active than the other isomers. The increases in ethoxyresorufin O-de-ethylase, n-hexane and benzo[a]pyrene hydroxylase activities were matched by elevated cytochrome P450 levels (Table 5.9).

Drug metabolising activity was also induced in the kidneys of these animals but, in the lung, xylene caused an inhibition of some enzymes. The overall effect on the body, however, is an increase in drug-metabolising capacity by induction of cytochrome P450 and, possibly, NADPH-cytochrome P450 reductase activity. The induction was similar to that found for phenobarbitone (see Chapter 3).

The aromatic hydrocarbons, therefore, seem to be phenobarbitone-like inducers of drug metabolism and are active by inhalation, thus indicating that workers in those industries using such solvents (e.g. the paint industry) may have induced drug metabolism as a result of solvent exposure.

Table 5.9 The effects of xylene and xylene isomers on hepatic drug metabolism in the rat

	Cytochrome P450	7-Ethoxyresorufin O-de-ethylase	n-Hexane 2-oxidation	Benzo[a]pyrene 4,5-hydroxylation
Xylene	190*	350*	480*	1000*
o-Xylene	175*	420*	820*	620*
m-Xylene	180*	370*	650*	1200*
p-Xylene	130*	150	450	450*

Results expressed as % vs control
* = $p < 0.05$
(Data from Toftgård, R. and Nilsen, O. (1982) *Toxicology* **23**, 197–212. Used with permission of the authors and Elsevier Science.)

The chlorinated hydrocarbons, in contrast to the aromatic hydrocarbons discussed above, do not always cause induction of drug metabolism. For example, trichloroethylene (the solvent often used in dry cleaning and fatty stain removal), when given chronically to rats, causes an increase in NADPH-cytochrome P450 reductase but a decrease in cytochrome P450 with a concomitant increase in aniline 4-hydroxylation and decrease in ethylmorphine N-demethylase. An increase in 4-nitrophenol glucuronidation was also seen. Some of these effects can be explained in terms of a direct effect of trichloroethylene on the liver enzymes. It is a 'suicide substrate' of cytochrome P450, i.e. it is metabolised by cytochrome P450 to an intermediate that destroys the enzyme. Trichloroethylene also competitively inhibits the metabolism of ethylmorphine when added into microsomal incubations and activates glucuronosyltransferase activity *in vitro*. The increase in aniline 4-hydroxylation is thought to be due to induction of specific forms of cytochrome P450, whereas overall cytochrome P450 levels fall. Trichloroethylene is, therefore, an unusual compound in that it simultaneously activates, inhibits, induces and destroys various drug metabolising enzyme activities.

Chloroform elicits similar effects to trichloroethylene, particularly with regard to the destruction of cytochrome P450, but dichloromethane, a close relative of chloroform, when administered to rats by inhalation, only causes induction of drug metabolism. There seems to be a dose-dependent induction of a number of enzyme activities, notably biphenyl 2-hydroxylation.

Chlorinated hydrocarbons can thus cause induction of drug metabolism in the same way as the aromatic hydrocarbons, but can also cause destruction of cytochrome P450 by acting as suicide substrates.

The ease of exposure to solvents (trichloroethylene is the solvent used for dry-cleaning fluids; toluene and xylene are the solvents in some adhesives) means that many people are subjected to the effects noted above, and this should be considered as a serious environmental problem.

5.2.2.3 Polychlorinated biphenyls (PCBs)
The polychlorinated biphenyls (PCBs) are a large group of compounds used in various manufacturing industries. Structurally the compounds can be split into two distinct groups: the planar and non-planar types (Figure 5.12).

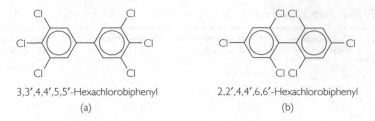

3,3′,4,4′,5,5′-Hexachlorobiphenyl   2,2′,4,4′,6,6′-Hexachlorobiphenyl
(a)   (b)

Figure 5.12 The structures of (a) planar and (b) non-planar polychlorinated biphenyls.

The 3,4,5-chloro-derivatives are planar whereas steric hindrance keeps the rings in the 2,4,6-chloro-derivatives at right angles to each other. These two groups of compound have different effects on drug metabolism. The planar PCBs induce hepatic drug metabolism similar to polycyclic hydrocarbons whereas the non-planar PCBs exhibit induction of drug metabolism of the phenobarbitone type.

Mixtures of PCBs (called Clophen A-50 or Arochlor-1254) induce cytochrome P450, NADPH-cytochrome P450 reductase, 4-nitroanisole O-demethylase, epoxide hydrolase and UDP-glucuronosyltransferase activities in rats within 1 week of the start of treatment. The overall induction pattern is typical of a mixed type of induction (probably due to both planar and non-planar isomers being present in the mixture). The induction of cytochrome P450 1A1 is particularly well established for Arochlor-1254 and appears to work via interaction with the Ah receptor. The point of interest is that a single dose of PCBs can maintain the induced level of enzymes for at least 1 month, indicating that these substances persist for long periods of time in the body.

5.2.3 Pesticides

Pesticides of various types are prevalent environmental contaminants in air, water and food. Again, there are many different chemical types of herbicides, insecticides, etc., and only a few will be discussed here with respect to their effects on drug metabolism. The compounds to be discussed are mirex, kepone, malathion, parathion and DDT.

Mirex and kepone are structurally similar insecticides. The effects of these compounds on the drug-metabolising capacity of rats is shown in Table 5.10. There is an indication that both of these compounds are specific inducing agents, differing from each other and from the classical enzyme inducers phenobarbitone and 3-methylcholanthrene.

Malathion and parathion are well-known, phosphothionate-type insecticides which are converted *in vivo* and *in vitro* to the corresponding phosphates, malaoxon and paraoxon. These insecticides are inhibitors of drug metabolism both *in vivo* and *in vitro*, probably due to competitive inhibition of the cytochrome P450-dependent reaction that also metabolises the insecticides.

Pesticides can, therefore, be inducers or inhibitors of drug metabolism. Their widespread use and persistence in the environment and in the body make them potentially important in determining drug metabolism both in man and in wild and domestic animals.

Table 5.10 Effects of mirex, kepone, 3-methylcholanthrene (3-MC) and phenobarbitone (PB) on hepatic drug metabolism

Inducing agent	Cytochrome P450 (nmoles mg^{-1} protein)	Biphenyl 4-hydroxylation (nmoles product min^{-1} mg^{-1} protein)	Biphenyl 2-hydroxylation (pmoles product min^{-1} mg^{-1} protein)	S-Warfarin 6-hydroxylation (pmoles product min^{-1} mg^{-1} protein)
Control	1.07 ± 0.01	0.54 ± 0.02	39 ± 2	0.13 ± 0.02
Mirex	1.77 ± 0.21**	0.56 ± 0.01	66 ± 1***	0.23 ± 0.02**
Kepone	1.95 ± 0.05**	0.55 ± 0.06	56 ± 14*	0.08 ± 0.02
3-MC	1.98 ± 0.17**	0.61 ± 0.03	232 ± 6***	0.18 ± 0.01**
PB				0.07 ± 0.01

Results expressed as: mean ± (standard error); * = $p < 0.05$; ** = $p < 0.01$; *** = $p < 0.001$.
(From Kaminsky, L.S. et al. (1978) Tox. Appl. Pharm. **43**, 327–338.)

5.2.4 Motor vehicle exhaust

Similar to tobacco smoke, the exhaust from a two-stroke petrol engine contains thousands of compounds including alkanes and cyclic hydrocarbons such as benzene, toluene and xylene as well as polycyclic aromatic hydrocarbons. It is little surprise that this potent mixture can induce drug metabolism. Inhalation of motor cycle exhaust led to a more than 30-fold induction of 7-ethoxyresorufin O-de-ethylase activity (with concomitant increase in CYP1A1) in rat liver. Similar increases in activity were seen in kidney and lung tissue.

5.3 RELATIVE IMPORTANCE OF PHYSIOLOGICAL AND ENVIRONMENTAL FACTORS IN DETERMINING DRUG-METABOLISING CAPACITY IN THE HUMAN POPULATION

As has been seen in the last two chapters, there are numerous factors that can affect the way in which the body handles drugs, varying from the genetic make-up of the person to how much grilled fish they eat. Attempts have been made to ascertain how much of the (sometimes quite large) inter-individual variations in drug metabolism are due to genetic differences and how much to environmental factors. Two opposing views – almost diametrically opposite to each other – have been put forward. The twin and family studies discussed earlier (see Chapter 4) seem to show that most, if not all, of the differences in drug metabolism in the population are due to genetic differences. Other research has indicated, by statistical analysis of family groups, that all of the inter-individual variations can be accounted for by environmental factors (alcohol, tea and coffee consumption and tobacco smoking), although the sex of the person has been included as an environmental factor.

Genetic sub-populations with respect to drug metabolism certainly exist (e.g. isoniazid 'fast' and 'slow' acetylators, and debrisoquine 'poor' and 'extensive' metabolisers (indicating differences in CYP2D6)) and so a genetic component of control of drug metabolism cannot be denied. The influence of environmental factors, on top of these obvious genetic differences, then lead to the inter-individual differences seen in the general population. The different research groups probably pick up different influences by virtue of the different substrates used, different experimental procedures and methods of statistical analysis. Antipyrine metabolism, for instance, may be mainly controlled by environmental factors, while debrisoquine metabolism is mainly genetically controlled.

The control of drug metabolism is, thus, an extremely complex subject with many controlling factors, some of which are interactive. A comprehensive summary of the subject is impossible but it is hoped that this chapter, together with Chapter 4, has given some idea of the factors involved and has stimulated the reader into further examination of one or more aspects of the subject, to which end a further reading list is included below.

FURTHER READING

Alvan, G. (1992) Genetic polymorphisms in drug metabolism. *J. Int. Med.* **231**, 571–573.

Ameer, B. and Weintraub, A. (1997) Drug interactions with grapefruit juice. *Clin. Pharmacokin.* **33**, 102–121.

Anderson, K.E. (1988) Influence of diet and nutrition on clinical pharmacokinetics. *Clin. Pharmacokin.* **14**, 325–346.

Azri, S. and Renton, K.W. (1991) Factors involved in the depression of hepatic mixed function oxidase during infection with Listeria monocytogenes. *Int. J. Immunopharmacol.* **13**, 197–204.

Berthou, F. *et al.* (1992) Interspecies variation in caffeine metabolism related to cytochrome P4501A enzymes. *Xenobiotica* **22**, 671–680.

Besunder, J.B. *et al.* (1988) Principles of drug biodisposition in the neonate. *Clin. Pharmacokin.* **14**, 189–216.

Burchell, B. and Coughtrie, M.W.H. (1997) Genetic and environmental factors associated with variations of human xenobiotic glucuronidation and sulphation. *Environ. Health Perspec.* **105**, 739–747.

Daly, A. (1999) Pharmacogenetics. In: *Handbook of Drug Metabolism* (T.F. Woolf, ed.). Marcel Dekker, New York, pp 131–145.

Dutton, G.J. (1978) Developmental aspects of drug conjugation, with special reference to glucuronidation. *Ann. Rev. Pharmacol. Toxicol.* **18**, 17–36.

Eichelbaum, M. and Gross, A.S. (1990) The genetic polymorphism of debrisoquine/sparteine metabolism – clinical aspects. *Pharmacol. Ther.* **46**, 377–394.

Gonzalez, F.J. and Meyer, U.A. (1991) Molecular genetics of the debrisoquine/sparteine polymorphism. *Clin. Pharmacol. Ther.* **50**, 233–238.

Guengerich, F.P. (1997) Comparisons of catalytic selectivity of cytochrome P450 subfamily enzymes from different species. *Chemico-Biol. Interact.* **106**, 161–182.

Hadidi, H. *et al.* (1999) Pharmacogenetics and toxicological consequences of human drug oxidation and reduction. In: *General and Applied Toxicology* 2nd edn, vol. 1 (B. Ballantyne *et al.*, eds). Macmillan Press, London, pp 215–250.

Horbach, G.J.M.J. *et al.* (1992) The effect of age on inducibility of various types of rat liver cytochrome P450. *Xenobiotica* **22**, 515–522.

Huupponen, R. *et al*. (1991) Activity of xenobiotic metabolizing liver enzymes in Zucker rats. *Res. Comm. Chem. Pathol. Pharmacol.* **72**, 307–314.

Idle, J.R. and Smith, R.L. (1979) Polymorphisms of oxidation at carbon centres of drugs and their clinical significance. *Drug Metab. Rev.* **9**, 301–318.

Jansen, P.L.M. (1996) Genetic diseases of bilirubin metabolism: the inherited unconjugated hyperbilirubinemias. *J. Hepatol.* **25**, 398–404.

Johnson, J.A. and Burlew, B.S. (1992) Racial differences in propranolol pharmacokinetics. *Clin. Pharmacol. Ther.* **51**, 495–500.

Kalow, W. (1992) *Pharmacogenetics of Drug Metabolism*. Pergamon Press, New York.

Kroemer, H.K. and Klotz, U. (1992) Glucuronidation of drugs. *Clin. Pharmacokin.* **23**, 292–310.

Ladona, M.G. *et al*. (1991) Differential foetal development of the *O*- and *N*-demethylation of codeine and dextromethorphan in man. *Br. J. Clin. Pharmacol.* **32**, 295–302.

Lavrijsen, K. *et al*. (1992) Comparative metabolism of flunarizine in rats, dogs and man: an in vitro study with subcellular liver fractions and isolated hepatocytes. *Xenobiotica* **22**, 815–836.

Lewis, D.F.V. (1998) The CYP2 family: models, mutants and interactions. *Xenobiotica* **28**, 617–661.

Lin, K-M. *et al*. (1996) The evolving science of pharmacogenetics: clinical and ethnic perspectives. *Psychopharm. Bull.* **32**, 205–217.

Longo, V. *et al*. (1991) Drug-metabolizing enzymes in liver, olfactory and respiratory epithelium of cattle. *J. Biochem. Toxicol.* **6**, 123–128.

Lou, Y.C. (1990) Differences in drug metabolism polymorphism between Orientals and Caucasians. *Drug Metab. Rev.* **22**, 451–475.

Masimirembwa, C.M. and Hasler, J.A. (1997) Genetic polymorphism of drug metabolising enzymes in African populations: implications for the use of neuroleptics and antidepressants. *Brain Res. Bull.* **44**, 561–571.

Meyer, U.A. and Zanger, U.M. (1997) Molecular mechanisms of genetic polymorphisms of drug metabolism. *Ann. Rev. Pharmacol. Toxicol.* **37**, 269–296.

Morgan, E.T. (1997) Regulation of cytochromes P450 during inflammation and infection. *Drug Metab. Rev.* **29**, 1129–1188.

Morgan, E.T. *et al*. (1998) Physiological and pathophysiological regulation of cytochrome P450. *Drug Metab. Disp.* **26**, 1232–1240.

Mugford, C.A. and Kedderis, G.L. (1998) Sex-dependent metabolism of xenobiotics. *Drug Metab. Rev.* **30**, 441–498.

Nagata, K. and Yamazoe, Y. (2000) Pharmacogenetics of sulphotransferase. *Ann. Rev. Pharmacol. Toxicol.* **40**, 159–176.

Ohmori, S. *et al*. (1991) Decrease in the specific forms of cytochrome P450 in liver microsomes of a mutant strain of rat with hyperbilirubinuria. *Res. Comm. Chem. Pathol. Pharmacol.* **72**, 243–253.

Puga, A. *et al*. (1997) Genetic polymorphisms in human drug-metabolizing enzymes: potential uses of reverse genetics to identify genes of toxicological relevance. *Crit. Rev. Toxicol.* **27**, 1990–2220.

Runge-Morris, M.A. (1997) Regulation of expression of the rodent cytosolic sulphotransferases. *FASEB J.* **11**, 109–117.

Scavone, J.M. *et al*. (1990) Differential effect of cigarette smoking on antipyrine oxidation and acetaminophen conjugation. *Pharmacology* **40**, 77–84.

Schmucker, D.L. *et al*. (1990) Effect of age and gender on *in vitro* properties of human liver microsomal monooxygenases. *Clin. Pharmacol. Ther.* **48**, 365–374.

Sim, E. and Hickman, D. (1991) Polymorphism in human N-acetyltransferase – the case of the missing allele. *TIPS* **12**, 211–213.

Skett, P. (1988) Biochemical basis of sex differences in drug metabolism. *Pharmacol. Ther.* **38**, 269–304.

Skett, P. and Gustafsson, J.-Å. (1979) Imprinting of enzyme systems of xenobiotic and steroid metabolism. *Rev. Biochem. Toxicol.* **1**, 27–52.

Smith, D.A. (1998) Human cytochromes P450: selectivity and measurement *in vivo*. *Xenobiotica* **28**, 1095–1128.

Smith, G. *et al.* (1998) Molecular genetics of the human cytochrome P450 monooxygenase superfamily. *Xenobiotica* **28**, 1129–1165.

Srivastava, P. *et al.* (1991) Effect of *Plasmodium berghei* infection and chloroquine on the hepatic drug metabolizing system of mice. *Int. J. Parasitol.* **4**, 463–466.

Tanaka, E. (1999) Update: genetic polymorphisms of drug-metabolising enzymes. *J. Clin. Pharm. Ther.* **24**, 323–329.

Tuckey, R.H. and Strassburg, C.P. (2000) Human UDP-glucuronosyltransferases: Metabolism, expression and disease. *Ann. Rev. Pharmacol. Toxicol.* **40**, 581–616.

Van der Weide, J. and Steijns, L.S. (1999) Cytochrome P450 enzyme system: genetic polymorphisms and impact on clinical pharmacology. *Ann. Clin. Biochem.* **36**, 722–729.

Walter-Sack, I. and Klotz, U. (1996) Influence of diet and nutritional status on drug metabolism. *Clin. Pharmacokin.* **31**, 47–64.

Woodhouse, K. (1992) Drugs and the liver III. Ageing of the liver and the metabolism of drugs. *Biopharmaceut. Drug Disp.* **13**, 311–320.

A list of useful web sites is included at the end of Chapters 2 and 3.

6 PHARMACOLOGICAL AND TOXICOLOGICAL ASPECTS OF DRUG METABOLISM

LEARNING OBJECTIVES

At the end of this chapter, you should be able to:
- Appreciate that the metabolism of drugs may change their pharmacological or toxicological properties
- Give examples of pharmacological deactivation and activation
- Give examples of toxicological deactivation and activation
- Understand how metabolites contribute to mutagenesis, carcinogenesis, teratogenesis, pulmonary toxicity, neurotoxicity, hepatotoxicity and nephrotoxicity
- Discuss the importance of the balance of activating and deactivating enzymes in dictating the toxicological outcome to xenobiotic exposure

6.1 INTRODUCTION

In general, the intensity and duration of drug action is proportional to the concentration of the drug at the site of action and the length of time it remains there. Therefore any factor that effectively alters the drug concentration at the active site will result in a changed pharmacological response to the drug. As indicated in previous chapters, the processes of drug metabolism result in biotransformation of the drug to metabolites that are chemically different from the parent drug and would therefore be expected to have an altered affinity for the drug receptor. Thus the processes of drug metabolism change the structure of the drug and essentially result in the production of a different chemical that often is not recognised by the relevant receptor system, and hence results in little or no pharmacological response. In this case, drug metabolism results in *pharmacological deactivation*. In contrast to the above, many drugs are pharmacologically inert and absolutely require metabolism to express their pharmacological effect (termed pro-drugs). Therefore in this case, the process of drug metabolism results in *pharmacological activation*.

The above simplified picture is somewhat confounded by the fact that drug metabolites can also elicit additional biological responses that are unrelated to the pharmacological properties of the parent compound. For example, drug metabolism may result in a *change* of the pharmacological properties of the drug, enabling metabolites to interact with other receptor systems. In addition, many toxicological responses to drugs and chemicals can be rationalised by the unique biological toxicity of metabolites not shared by the parent compound, and is therefore an example of *toxicological activation*.

From the above discussion it is clear that the processes of drug metabolism have to be considered as a 'double-edged sword' in that, depending on the specific drug or chemical in question, a change in the pharmacology or toxicology of the drug may arise. Accordingly, it is the purpose of this chapter to consider the above concepts in more detail by examining the pharmacological and toxicological aspects of drug metabolism.

6.2 PHARMACOLOGICAL ASPECTS OF DRUG METABOLISM

The metabolism of a drug may alter the drug's pharmacological properties in one of several ways:

- Pharmacological deactivation
- Pharmacological activation
- Change in type of pharmacological response
- No change in pharmacological activity
- Change in drug uptake (absorption)
- Change in drug distribution
- Enterohepatic circulation.

6.2.1 Pharmacological deactivation

The concept of specific enzyme systems existing for the deactivation or detoxification of drugs is not novel. For example, many chemicals or metabolites that are produced during normal intermediary metabolism are potentially toxic to the organism and enzyme systems are present that facilitate their inactivation. This is clearly seen in the efficient detoxification of hydrogen peroxide (arising from oxidative metabolism of endogenous substrates) by enzymes such as catalase. In a similar manner, many therapeutically used drugs and other xenobiotics are inactivated by the phase 1 enzymes of drug metabolism due to the substantially reduced pharmacological activity of the metabolite as compared to the parent drug (Figure 6.1).

An interesting and specific example of the above concept is the cytochrome P450-dependent pharmacological inactivation of the anticoagulant drug, warfarin. In man, the major route of warfarin biotransformation is the hepatic CYP2C9-dependent hydroxylation of the parent compound at the 7-position (Figure 6.2). Since there is a narrow margin of clinical safety for this drug (i.e. a low therapeutic index), then it follows that the levels and activity of this cytochrome P4502C9 isoform crucially influence both the pharmacology and toxicology of this drug. As a related issue, it should be noted that warfarin can be metabolised at various positions in the molecule by different forms of cytochrome P450, further emphasising the importance of the tissue *complement* of cytochromes P450 in dictating the clinical response to drugs. As a further refinement of cytochrome P450 selectivity in drug biotransformation, warfarin exists in racemic (R and S) forms, each racemate exhibiting a different preference for regioselectivity of hydroxylation by the cytochrome P450 isoforms.

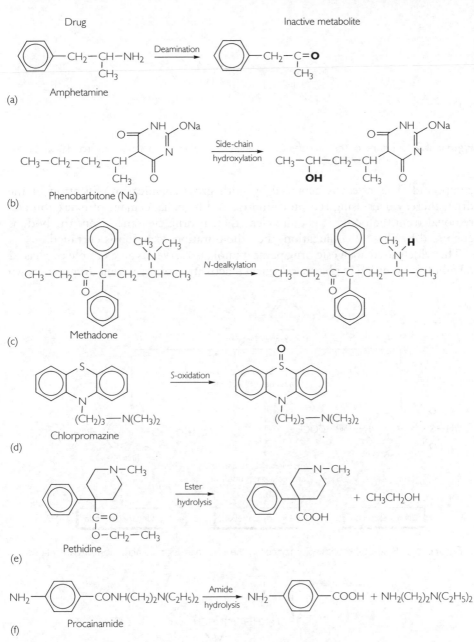

Figure 6.1 Role of phase I enzymes in the pharmacological inactivation of drugs.

It should be pointed out that the phase 2 conjugating enzymes play a very important role in the pharmacological inactivation of drugs and further inactivation of their phase 1 metabolites. Although a few exceptions are known, the majority of drug conjugates are pharmacologically less active than the parent

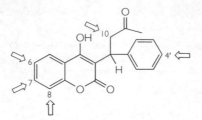

Figure 6.2 Structure of the anticoagulant warfarin and sites of metabolic hydroxylation by the cytochromes P450.

compound. This effect is achieved by both gross chemical modification of the drug, thereby decreasing receptor affinity, and by enhancement of excretion and removal from the body. It is quite clear that, if drug clearance from the body is enhanced by phase 2 conjugation, then the duration of action is curtailed.

The widely used analgesic drug paracetamol also serves as an example of phase 2 metabolism resulting in pharmacological inactivation of the parent drug. As shown

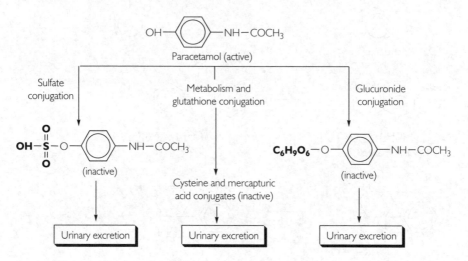

Figure 6.3 Role of the phase 2 enzymes in the pharmacological inactivation of paracetamol.

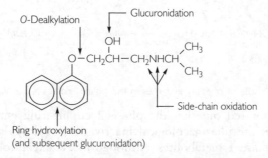

Figure 6.4 Metabolic pathways resulting in the pharmacological inactivation of propranolol.

in Figure 6.3, paracetamol undergoes glutathione, glucuronide and sulfate conjugation and the resulting phase 2 conjugates are pharmacologically inactive. However, an alternative metabolic pathway actually activates paracetamol to a toxic metabolite (*N*-acetyl-*p*-benzoquinoneimine, see later), again emphasising the importance of the *balance* of metabolic pathways dictating biological responses. Furthermore, many drugs are pharmacologically deactivated by simultaneous phase 1 and phase 2 metabolic attack at different positions in the molecule as is observed in the metabolic inactivation of the betablocker, propranolol (Figure 6.4).

6.2.2 Pharmacological activation

In contrast to the concepts discussed above, many drugs and chemicals absolutely require metabolic activation before they can exert their pharmacological action. This process of metabolic activation is usually associated with the phase 1 enzymes. Many of these parent drugs are essentially devoid of pharmacological activity and this has led to the development of the so-called pro-drugs. A classical example of pro-drug activation by metabolism was the early use of the dye prontosil in the 1930s to treat bacterial infections. *In vitro* studies clearly showed that prontosil itself was inactive and required metabolic azo reduction to liberate the pharmacologically active component, sulfanilamide (Figure 6.5).

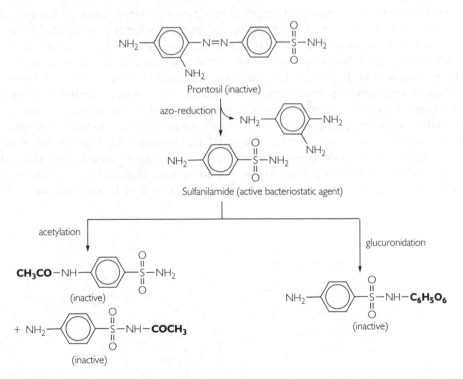

Figure 6.5 Role of metabolism in the pharmacological activation of prontosil and the pharmacological inactivation of its major metabolite, sulfanilamide.

It should be noted that the active sulfanilamide is subsequently metabolically inactivated by N-acetylation at both nitrogen atoms and by N-glucuronidation at the amide nitrogen. Accordingly, it is clear that the therapeutic effectiveness of this class of drugs is strongly influenced by the prevailing tissue balance of the azo reductase on the one hand and the N-acetyltransferase and glucuronidation enzymes on the other.

The above concept of pro-drug activation has been used to target drugs to their specific site of action. For example, the drug levodopa is metabolically activated in the neurone to dopamine, but the drug is given as the levodopa precursor due to its more facile uptake into the neurone. Dopamine does not cross the blood–brain barrier. Therefore, L-dopa is given as a precursor as it does cross the blood–brain barrier. In this context, it should be noted that carbidopa (a hydrazine derivative of dopamine and a *peripheral* dopa decarboxylase inhibitor) is often given in conjunction with L-dopa. The therapeutic rationale behind this combination therapy (frequently used in the treatment of Parkinsonism) is that carbidopa does not cross the blood–brain barrier and therefore does not interfere with the beneficial central effects of L-dopa. However, because carbidopa inhibits the peripheral formation of dopamine from L-dopa, the peripheral side effects of L-dopa are substantially diminished, thereby allowing a reduction in the therapeutically effective dose of L-dopa.

Another example of biotransformation resulting in pharmacological activation is in the clinical usage of mercaptopurine, a chemotherapeutic agent used in the treatment of patients with leukaemia. The clinical usefulness of mercaptopurine is limited by its rapid biotransformation by xanthine oxidase to the inactive metabolite, 6-thiouric acid. Because of this extensive metabolism, the drug has to be given in high doses, thereby predisposing the liver and other tissues to cellular damage and hence toxicity. The above clinical limitations can be largely overcome by administering mercaptopurine as its cysteine conjugate where advantage is taken of the fact that the anionic form of the pro-drug conjugate is selectively taken up by the renal organic anion transport system. The conjugate is subsequently cleaved by the kidney cysteine conjugate β-lyase enzyme system (Figure 6.6), thus creating a clinical use for this cysteine conjugate in the treatment of kidney tumours.

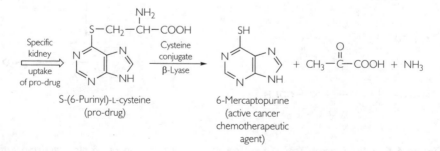

Figure 6.6 Kidney uptake and pharmacological activation of the prodrug, S-(6-purinyl)-L-cysteine.

Table 6.1 Drug metabolism reactions resulting in pharmacological activation

Pro-drug	Clinical use	Metabolic conversion	Active drug/metabolite
Azathioprine	Immunosuppressant	Thio-ether hydrolysis	Mercaptopurine
Chloral hydrate	Sedative/hypnotic	Reduction	Trichloroethanol
Clofibrate	Hypolipidaemic	Ester hydrolysis	Clofibric acid
Cyclophosphamide	Anti-tumour/immunosuppressant	Hydroxylation	4-Hydroxy-cyclophosphamide (precursor to other active metabolites)
Disulfiram	Alcohol withdrawal	Dithiol reduction	Diethylthiocarbamic acid
Glyceryl triacetate	Antifungal	Ester hydrolysis	Acetic acid
Methyldopa	Antihypertensive	Decarboxylation and hydroxylation	α-methylnoradrenaline
Prednisone	Anti-inflammatory	Keto reduction	Prednisolone
Primaquine	Antimalarial	Demethylation and oxidation	Primaquine quinone
Primidone	Anti-epileptic	Oxidation	Phenobarbitone
Proguanil	Antimalarial	Cyclization	Cycloguanil
Prontosil	Antibiotic	Azo-reduction	Sulfanilamide
Succinylsulfathiazole	Antibiotic	Amide hydrolysis	Sulfathiazole

There are many other examples of drugs whose metabolism results in pharmacological activation and some of these are given in Table 6.1.

6.2.3 Change in type of pharmacological response

In addition to modulating pharmacological responses in either a positive or negative manner as described above, the process of drug metabolism can also result in *a change* in the pharmacology of the parent compound. For example, iproniazid was formerly used as an anti-depressant, but has subsequently been removed from the market because it caused severe liver toxicity in man. Iproniazid is metabolised by N-dealkylation, resulting in the formation of the metabolite isoniazid which has pronounced anti-tubercular activity, a pharmacological activity not associated with the parent drug. Another example of this phenomenon is seen in the metabolism of the tricyclic anti-depressant drug imipramine. This drug undergoes an enzymatic N-demethylation reaction, resulting in the formation of desmethylimipramine, a compound that is substantially more potent than the parent drug as an inhibitor of the neuronal uptake of noradrenaline but less potent for the uptake of 5HT.

A third example of the ability of drug metabolism to result in a change in pharmacological response is seen in the metabolism of diazepam (Valium), a benzodiazepine chiefly used as a tranquilliser. The drug undergoes N-demethylation and subsequent ring hydroxylation, yielding oxazepam as a metabolite, the metabolite having pronounced anti-convulsant properties. The metabolic pathways involved in the above reactions are summarised in Figure 6.7.

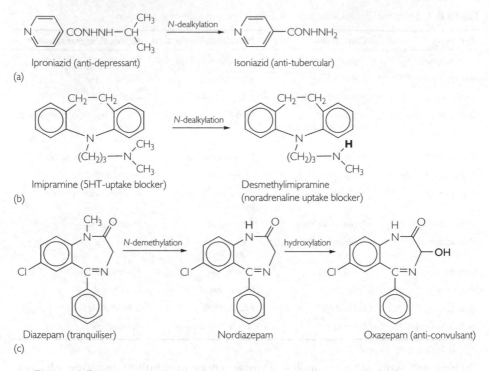

Figure 6.7 Drug metabolism resulting in a change in the type of pharmacological activity.

6.2.4 No change in pharmacological activity

Several drugs are metabolised to compounds that have the same or similar pharmacological activity. An example of this type is the N-deethylation of the local anaesthetic lignocaine. The N-deethylated metabolite (monoethylglycylxylidide) is as active as the parent compound and it would appear that metabolism serves no useful immediate purpose here. However, it should be emphasised that metabolism may prime the substrate for subsequent phase 2 reactions and indirectly facilitate drug excretion and hence termination of pharmacological activity.

6.2.5 Changes in drug uptake

Changes in drug uptake by metabolism may be seen after the oral administration of drugs and is dependent on the enzymes at the site of uptake, for example, the gastrointestinal tract. In most cases, drug metabolism at the site of uptake inhibits drug absorption as seen in the formation of sulfate conjugates of phenolic drugs after oral administration. As shown in Figure 6.8, isoprenaline sulfation and isoniazid acetylation by enzymes in the intestinal wall and gut flora result in more polar metabolites. The polar metabolites are less readily absorbed across the gut wall as compared to the parent drug and are consequently preferentially excreted in the faeces.

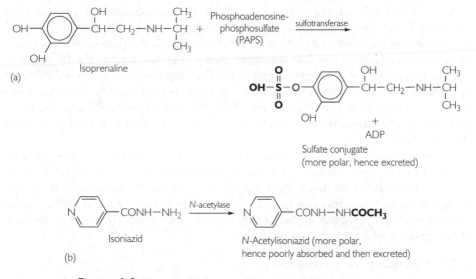

(a)

(b)

Figure 6.8 The role of drug metabolism in modifying drug uptake.

It is interesting to note that in certain cases the metabolism of a drug at the uptake site is an important factor in determining the most effective route of administration. For instance, in the example of the anti-asthmatic drug isoprenaline, given above, it is clear that oral administration is not an effective means of getting the drug to its site of action (lung) because of extensive gut metabolism. To get over this problem, isoprenaline may be given sublingually and absorbed through the buccal mucosa. Unfortunately, the circulating drug is rapidly inactivated (again by metabolism) in the liver. Isoprenaline is best administered via aerosol inhalation and, in this way, the inactivating metabolic pathways are by-passed and the drug directly reaches the lungs in sufficiently high concentration to be pharmacologically active.

In contrast to the above, gut metabolism can be used to advantage as in the oral administration of the 4-amino-substituted sulfonamide antibiotics such as succinylsulfathiazole. This drug is poorly absorbed through the gut wall and is readily hydrolysed by gut enzymes to the active sulfathiazole. This local hydrolysis in the gut ensures high, effective antibiotic concentrations, and is therefore very useful in the treatment of gut infections.

6.2.6 Changes in drug distribution

Drug distribution to the various tissues in the body (and hence the site of action) is dependent on several factors including the lipid solubility of the drug. A highly lipophilic drug will be localised in highest concentrations in tissues with high fat content such as adipose tissues and the brain. As metabolism causes drugs to be less lipid soluble in most cases, metabolism will then alter drug distribution away from the high-fat tissues and into the high water content tissues such as blood and the kidney.

A good example of the above concept is the distribution of the narcotic analgesic morphine. Morphine is highly lipophilic and is not readily excreted because it is quickly absorbed into lipid-rich tissues, including the brain. However, morphine undergoes phase 2 conjugation with glucuronic acid in the liver, forming the morphine-3-glucuronide metabolite. This metabolite is water-soluble and does not readily enter the brain and the conjugate is then rapidly excreted. Thus hepatic metabolism in this instance precludes the access of morphine to the brain and thereby diminishes the pharmacological response by redistribution away from the site of action.

The lipophilicity of drugs can also radically influence the rate of onset of drug action. For example, diamorphine (diacetylmorphine, or as it is better known, heroin) enters the brain much more rapidly than morphine because of its higher lipophilicity, and therefore has a more rapid onset of action. Once in the brain, the diamorphine is rapidly metabolised to morphine, whereupon the pharmacological effects (primarily analgesia) are observed.

6.2.7 Enterohepatic circulation

The specific route of drug excretion is largely influenced by its molecular weight. Drugs having a molecular weight of under approximately 300 are largely excreted in urine, whereas drugs with a higher molecular weight are mainly excreted in the bile and hence into the intestine. Once in the intestine, a drug glucuronide conjugate has two possible fates. It can either be excreted in the faeces or, additionally, the glucuronide conjugate can be hydrolysed back to the parent drug by the action of the enzyme β-glucuronidase which is present in gut bacteria. The free, de-conjugated drug is then re-absorbed through the gut wall and re-enters the liver via the hepatic portal vein. The free drug can then be re-conjugated with glucuronic acid, secreted into the bile and then intestine and the cyclic process starts again. This cycling of a drug is known as the enterohepatic circulation and is summarised in Chapter 2 (Figure 2.19). The above recirculation of drugs can take place for several cycles and the overall result is that the drug is retained in the body and has a substantially increased half-life. Provided that the drug concentration is maintained high enough at the site of action, it is quite clear that this metabolism-based cycle can result in a prolongation of pharmacological activity, as is seen in the example given for chloramphenicol (Figure 6.9). The eventual excretion of the drug then arises from the faecal excretion of drug conjugate that escapes hydrolysis in the intestine during each turn of the cycle and by other metabolic pathways.

It would appear that drugs get trapped in this cycle by accident rather than design. It is well known that conjugates of endogenous compounds such as steroids, bile salts and bilirubin undergo the same enterohepatic circulation, and therefore drugs are 'ensnared' in a normal physiological process, which is designed to salvage important endogenous compounds.

In conclusion, drug metabolism can profoundly alter the uptake, distribution and pharmacological action of a particular drug as well as direct its excretion pattern. In addition, drug metabolism is of major importance in determining the method of administration and on deciding the correct dose and frequency of drug delivery.

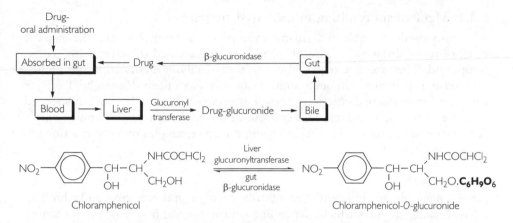

Figure 6.9 Enterohepatic circulation of drugs.

In fact, apart from the inherent pharmacological activity of the drug itself, the metabolism of a drug is probably the most important consideration to be made in drug design and therapeutics.

6.3 TOXICOLOGICAL ASPECTS OF XENOBIOTIC METABOLISM

At this point it is instructive to put our overall knowledge of drug and chemical toxicity into perspective, such that we can appreciate the overall contribution made by biotransformation reactions. It may surprise the reader to learn that, in terms of all the chemicals (including drugs) in use today, we know less about their toxicity than we have knowledge thereof (Table 6.2). Although the remainder of this chapter places emphasis on well-documented examples of the role of biotransformation in drug and xenobiotic toxicity, it must be borne in mind that the above lack of toxicity information may obscure a far greater prominence for metabolism than we are currently aware of.

As discussed above for the pharmacological properties of drugs and their metabolites, drug metabolism can result in either a decreased or increased toxicity of the parent compound, depending, of course, on the inherent biological potencies (toxicities) of the drug and its metabolite(s).

Table 6.2 Toxicity assessment information available

	Percentage toxicity information available		
	Complete	Partial	None
Drugs	18	50	32
Pesticides	8	54	38
Food additives	4	50	46
Cosmetics	2	51	47
Chemicals	16	6	78

6.3.1 Metabolism resulting in increased toxicity

As summarised in Table 6.3, many examples are known where the hepatic metabolism of drugs and chemicals results in an increased toxicity of the parent compound. The enzymes responsible for this metabolic toxification are mainly the phase 1 enzymes. Although some examples have been documented on the participation of phase 2 reactions, these latter enzymes are more often associated with detoxification reactions. This concept of metabolic toxification can be amply demonstrated by considering the following specific examples of toxic reactions to drugs and chemicals.

Mutagenesis
Many chemicals are inherently chemically reactive and can covalently bind to DNA, forming adducts which, depending on the specific nature of the mutation, are a common prelude to xenobiotic-induced cancer. However, many drugs and chemicals have a low mutagenic potential *per se* and require metabolic activation to express their mutagenicity, i.e. the metabolite is the directly acting mutagen. This is clearly seen in the most commonly used *in vitro* test for mutagenicity, namely the Ames test using the bacterium *Salmonella typhimurium* as the genetic indicator. This bacterial system is augmented by the addition of inducer-pretreated liver homogenates from various species, which serve as a source of drug-metabolising enzymes to activate the pre-mutagen. Examples of mutagens which require metabolic activation (mainly by the cytochromes P450) are benzo[a]pyrene, dimethylnitrosamine and 1,2-dimethylhydrazine, amongst many others.

Genotoxic carcinogenesis
Chemically-induced liver tumours can arise in the hepatocyte (liver adenomas and primary hepatocellular carcinoma), the hepatic vasculature (hemangiosarcoma) or the bile duct (cholangiosarcoma) and there are several reasonably well documented cases where metabolism plays a necessary and pivotal role.

Aflatoxin B_1 is an extremely potent liver carcinogen (induced by μg doses) derived from fungally contaminated peanuts in the tropics and is very likely a human carcinogen, although the coexistence of hepatitis B obscures a realistic

Table 6.3 Metabolism resulting in increased toxicity of drugs and chemicals

Compound	Metabolic pathway	Toxicity
2-Acetylaminofluorene	N-Hydroxylation and sulfation	Hepatocarcinogenesis
Benzene	Epoxidation (and other pathways leading to ring opening)	Aplastic anaemia/leukaemia
Cyclophosphamide	Hydroxylation (and rearrangement)	Teratogenesis
Halothane	Defluorination	Hepatitis
Isoniazid	Acetylation and hydrolysis	Hepatic necrosis
Methoxyflurane	Defluorination	Nephrotoxicity

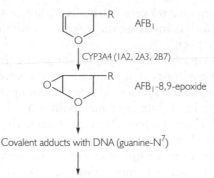

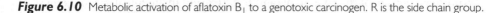

Figure 6.10 Metabolic activation of aflatoxin B₁ to a genotoxic carcinogen. R is the side chain group.

assessment of the epidemiological data. Aflatoxin is metabolised by CYP1A2, CYP2A3, CYP2B7 and CYP3A4 in man to produce the DNA-reactive 8,9-epoxide metabolite, forming aflatoxin B_1–N^7-guanine adducts which may be excreted in the urine (Figure 6.10). The chemically reactive epoxide may alternatively be detoxified by epoxide hydrolase and/or the glutathione *S*-transferases. It is interesting to note that these latter two enzymes are polymorphically expressed in the human population and a genetic lack of these enzymes may predispose these subpopulations to be relatively sensitive to the hepatocarcinogenicity of aflatoxin B_1.

Vinyl chloride is a high-volume industrial chemical extensively used in plastics manufacture (polyvinyl chloride, PVC), as a refrigerant and in adhesives and therefore has a substantial potential for occupational and environmental exposure to man. Vinyl chloride is a proven human carcinogen, producing a rare hemangiosarcoma (developed from the epithelial cells of the hepatic sinusoids) which is absolutely dependent on bioactivation by several cytochromes P450. The reactive metabolite is chloroethylene oxide (Figure 6.11) which forms N^7-guanine, adenine and cytosine adducts in DNA. Interestingly, the reactive metabolite is formed in

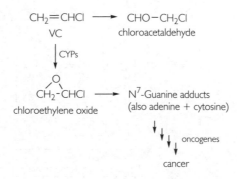

Figure 6.11 Role of cytochrome P450 in the metabolic activation of vinyl chloride (VC) to a hepatocarcinogen.

the parenchymal (hepatocyte) cells in the liver, but not in the target endothelial cells of the sinusoid, thus invoking the distinct possibility of reactive metabolite transport within the liver.

As discussed previously, the polycyclic aromatic hydrocarbons represent a ubiquitous group of environmental pollutants that are well documented in causing cancer in many mammalian species. The parent compounds are relatively innocuous and chemically inert, but their metabolites are biologically active and are potent carcinogens. The polycyclic aromatic hydrocarbons are metabolised by the cytochromes P450 and epoxide hydrolase, forming the electrophilic diol-epoxide metabolites which are then capable of covalent binding to nucleic acids and hence the initiation of chemical carcinogenesis (see Figure 2.17 for the metabolic pathways involved).

Another example of the role of metabolic activation in chemical carcinogenesis is the metabolism of the compound 2-acetylaminofluorene. This synthetic compound was originally intended for use as an insecticide, and during routine safety studies prior to introduction to the market, it was discovered that it was an extremely potent hepatocarcinogen. Further studies on this carcinogen have amply documented the fact that both phase 1 (cytochromes P450) and phase 2 enzymes (the sulfotransferases) are involved in the bioactivation of this carcinogen (Figure 6.12). The sulfation of N-hydroxy-acetylaminofluorene by the sulfotransferase enzymes plays a critical role in determining hepatotoxicity. As can be seen in Table 6.4, there is a pronounced species/sex sensitivity to N-hydroxy-acetylaminofluorene, in that the male rat is very sensitive, the male guinea pig is resistant and the female rat

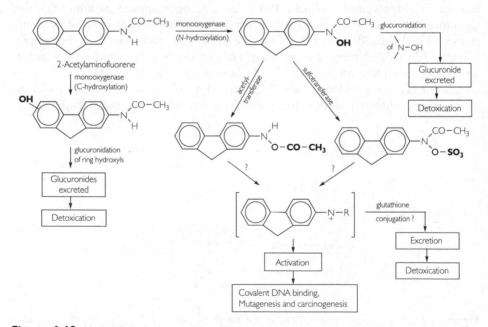

Figure 6.12 Metabolic activation and inactivation of the hepatocarcinogen, 2-acetylaminofluorene.

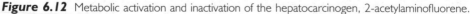

Table 6.4 Species differences in sulfotransferase activity and the relationship to hepatotoxicity

Species + sex	Liver SULT activity (units)	Covalent binding (units)	N—OH AAF hepatocarcinogenicity
Rat (M)	23	38	+++++
Rat (F)	4	4	+
G.pig (M)	<0.3	<0.5	−

somewhere in between. This is related to the fact that the most sensitive species (male rat) expresses a high level of sulfotransferase activity, which is related to covalent binding and (presumably) hepatocarcinogenicity.

The importance of the drug-metabolising enzymes in many types of chemical carcinogenesis cannot be overemphasised and, in addition to the above examples, many other chemicals (including the aromatic amines and nitrosamines) are dependent on metabolism for expression of their carcinogenicity. As a caveat to the above general description, it must be borne in mind that metabolism alone is not the sole determinant of carcinogenicity of drugs and chemicals – many other factors are important for expression of carcinogenicity including the ability to repair genotoxic lesions, promotion and cancer progression and genetic predisposition. However, this is a large and complex area outside the scope of this discussion.

Teratogenesis
Several drugs and chemicals are known to interfere with the processes of embryo development and, if given at the critical stage of organogenesis, can result in malformations of the embryo (teratogenesis). The anti-tumour drug cyclophosphamide is a well-documented teratogen and several studies have shown that the metabolites of cyclophosphamide are much more teratogenic than the parent compound. As shown in Figure 6.13, cyclophosphamide undergoes cytochrome P450-dependent hydroxylation at the 4-position and this hydroxylated metabolite serves as the precursor for the toxic metabolites acrolein and phosphoramide mustard. Although it is not known with any degree of certainty which of these two metabolites of cyclophosphamide is the major teratogen, it is quite clear that metabolism is a prerequisite for the expression of cyclophosphamide teratogenicity.

Pulmonary toxicity
The lung is a complex organ consisting of over 40 different cell types. Several drug-metabolising enzymes are expressed in the lung (particularly the non-ciliated bronchiolar epithelial cell, otherwise known as the Clara cell), including CYPs 1A1, 2B6, 2E1, 2F1, 3A4 and 4B1 and phase 2 enzymes, albeit at a lower level than in the liver. Several chemicals cause pulmonary toxicity and examples where metabolism is required are given in Table 6.5, some of which will now be considered in more detail.

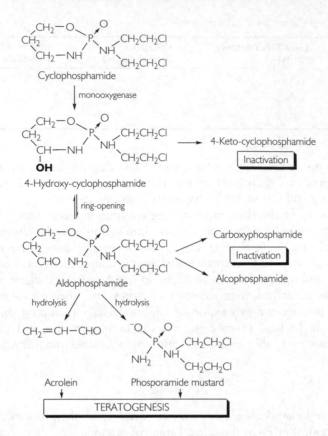

Figure 6.13 Metabolic activation of the teratogen cyclophosphamide.

Table 6.5 Role of bioactivation in the pulmonary toxicity of xenobiotics

Xenobiotic	Activating enzymes	Type of toxicity
4-Ipomeanol	P450	Clara cell necrosis
3-Methylfuran	P450	Clara cell necrosis
Benzo[a]pyrene	P450, EH	Carcinoma
Thiourea	P450, FMO	Type I cell damage
Naphthalene	P450	Clara cell necrosis
Nitrofurantoin	P450 reductase, XO	Fibrosis
Paraquat	P450 reductase	Necrosis + oedema
Parathion	P450	Oedema
Carbon tetrachloride	P450	Clara/Type II necrosis
Hydrazines	MAO	Carcinoma

Abbreviations used: P450, cytochrome P450; EH, epoxide hydrolase; FMO, flavin monooxygenase; XO, xanthine oxidase; MAO, monoamine oxidase.

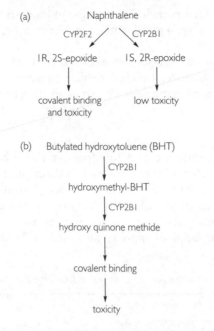

(a) Naphthalene

CYP2F2 / \ CYP2B1

1R, 2S-epoxide   1S, 2R-epoxide

covalent binding   low toxicity
and toxicity

(b) Butylated hydroxytoluene (BHT)

↓ CYP2B1

hydroxymethyl-BHT

↓ CYP2B1

hydroxy quinone methide

↓

covalent binding

↓

toxicity

Figure 6.14 Role of cytochromes P450 in the metabolic activation of (a) naphthalene and (b) butylated hydroxytoluene to pulmonary toxins.

Naphthalene (an industrial chemical) and butylated hydroxytoluene (a food antioxidant) both produce reactive metabolites produced by the cytochromes P450, which result in covalent binding to critical macromolecular targets in the cell, leading to pulmonary toxicity (Figure 6.14).

4-Ipomeanol, a furan derivative found on mouldy sweet potatoes, produces a characteristic pulmonary toxicity in several mammalian species (necrosis of the non-ciliated bronchiolar epithelial or Clara cells). Current evidence suggests that 4-ipomeanol is metabolised by a specific pulmonary cytochrome P450, resulting in the formation of a highly biological reactive intermediate. This intermediate covalently binds to critical macromolecular targets in the Clara cell, resulting in the observed necrosis in this cell type. It is interesting to note that 4-ipomeanol is selectively toxic to the lung and is relatively non-toxic to the liver, an organ very rich in xenobiotic metabolising enzymes. This apparent contradiction may be rationalised by the observation that the liver lacks the appropriate form of cytochrome P450 necessary for activation or that the liver is well-endowed with the detoxifying phase 2 enzymes that remove the reactive intermediate.

The herbicide paraquat is a very toxic compound, as demonstrated by the many accidental deaths in humans, particularly young children. Paraquat appears to 'hijack' the specific pulmonary uptake mechanism for polyamines, thus concentrating this chemical in the lung, particularly the Type I and Type II cells, the site of toxicity. The resultant pulmonary toxicity of paraquat is therefore due to a combination of several factors including specific pulmonary uptake, redox cycling and generation of toxic oxygen metabolites and perturbation of redox homeostasis in this tissue.

The above discussion emphasises the importance of metabolism in producing toxic metabolites. Furthermore, it is clear that the presence (or absence) of phase 1 and phase 2 enzymes is an important determinant of selective organ toxicity of drugs and chemicals.

Hepatic toxicity

The liver is quite frequently a target for drug- and xenobiotic-induced toxicity and a summary of the factors that predispose this tissue are given in Table 6.6, and examples of hepatic toxicants are given in Table 6.7. A well documented example of a hepatotoxin is paracetamol, which in high doses produces hepatic necrosis in both experimental animals and man. Paracetamol is an analgesic and antipyretic drug which is safe in the range of approximately 0.5–3.0 g/day. However, signs of

Table 6.6 Factors predisposing the liver to chemical-induced hepatotoxicity

- Large organ, 2% of body weight in man
- First tissue to receive chemicals absorbed from gut
- Extensive blood supply: 80% from portal vein and 25% from hepatic artery
- Different cell types including hepatocytes (90% of parenchyma volume), sinusoid endothelial cells, Kupffer cells and Ito cells
- Supports many biochemical functions, perturbation of which may lead to toxicity
- Expresses high levels of drug metabolising enzymes, almost all of which are induced/inhibited by xenobiotics
- Substantial capacity for self-repair, but can be overwhelmed
- Normally a quiescent organ but cell division readily happens

Table 6.7 Hepatotoxic agents

Type of toxicity	Example
Acute liver necrosis	CCl_4, paracetamol
Acute hepatocellular hepatitis	Isoniazid, halothane
Macrovacuolar steatosis	Valproate, ethanol
Chronic-active hepatitis	Nitrofurantoin
Phospholipidosis	Perhexiline, amiodarone
Fatty liver	Ethanol, 1,2-dimethylformamide
Cirrhosis	Ethanol, arsenic
Cholestasis	Anabolic steroids, chlorpromazine
Portal hypertension	Vinyl chloride, arsenic
Veno-occlusive disease	Pyrrolizidine alkaloids
Liver vein thrombosis	Hormonal contraceptives
Liver tumours	Vinyl chloride, aflatoxin B_1

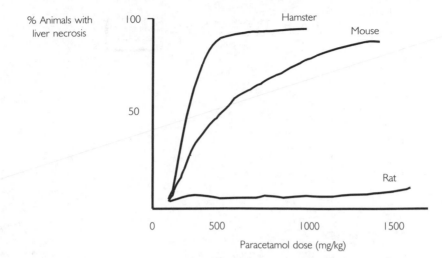

Figure 6.15 Species differences in susceptibility to paracetamol-induced liver necrosis.

intoxication are seen at 4–10 g/day in sensitive individuals and over 10 g/day will almost certainly produce liver toxicity (and kidney complications) in the majority of the population.

Paracetamol-induced liver toxicity is characterised by centrilobular necrosis and fulminant liver damage, accompanied by renal damage and failure. As shown in Figure 6.15, there is a pronounced species sensitivity to paracetamol toxicity, with the hamster being particularly sensitive, the rat being effectively resistant and the mouse intermediary. Furthermore, the severity of toxicity is increased/decreased by cytochrome P450 inducers/inhibitors respectively, thereby implicating a role for an active metabolite. This indeed turned out to be the case and, as shown in Figure 6.16, the active metabolite has been identified as N-acetyl-p-benzoquinoneimine. The degree of hepatic necrosis correlates reasonably well with covalent binding of N-acetyl-p-benzoquinoneimine (or a very similar rearrangement product) which is thought to initiate the cellular events leading to frank hepatic toxicity. However, the precise molecular and cellular mechanisms of toxicity still remain a topic of debate and are outside the scope of this text. Specifically, CYP2E1 (ethanol-inducible) appears to be the major form of cytochrome P450 responsible for N-acetyl-p-benzoquinoneimine formation, via an initial N-hydroxylation event, as clearly substantiated by the lack of paracetamol liver toxicity in CYP2E1-knockout mice (where the CYP2E1 has been entirely deleted), although CYPs 1A1, 1A2 and 3A4 may also play a role. It is indeed ironic that ethanol induces CYP2E1 (and therefore increases N-acetyl-p-benzoquinoneimine formation), considering how frequently paracetamol is taken the 'morning after' a substantial encounter with ethanol, further emphasised by the increased frequency of paracetamol-induced liver damage in alcoholics. Figure 6.16 also highlights a crucial and protective role for glutathione in protecting the liver, as it can conjugate the reactive imine metabolite and hence result in detoxification. This is taken

189

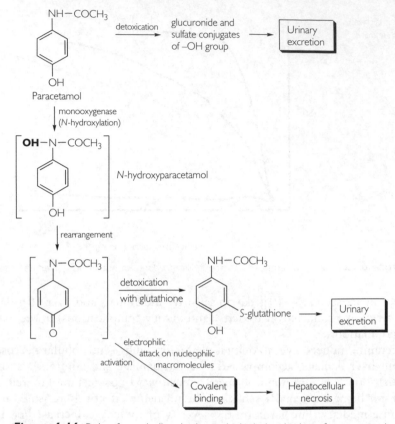

Figure 6.16 Role of metabolism in the toxicological activation of paracetamol.

advantage of in the clinical treatment of paracetamol overdosage, where N-acetyl cysteine (a glutathione precursor) can help protect against the liver toxicity.

There is substantial variation in susceptibility to paracetamol-induced liver damage in the human population, thought to be due to differences in the expression/polymorphism of CYP2E1. Approximately 5–10% of the human population form the reactive metabolite at a rate similar to the hamster/mouse (susceptible) and therefore would constitute an at-risk sub-population.

Carbon tetrachloride (CCl$_4$) is probably one of the most intensively studied liver toxicants and produces acute centrilobular necrosis and fatty liver, followed by chronic effects including cirrhosis and liver tumours in susceptible species. Again, after covalent binding/lipid peroxidation, biotransformation plays a role in toxicity as mediated by cytochrome P450-mediated *reductive* metabolism to the key trichloromethyl radical, as shown in Figure 6.17. Radical formation is produced in a reductive mode by CYPs 2B1 and 2E1 and results in covalent binding and the initiation of cytotoxic lipid peroxidation. Again, much work has been done on investigating the specific molecular/cellular events that subsequently occur, and the interested reader is referred to the bibliography at the end of this chapter.

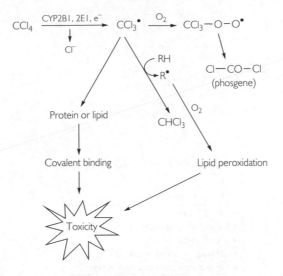

Figure 6.17 Reductive bioactivation of carbon tetrachloride and liver toxicity. RH represents a polyunsaturated fatty acid.

Nephrotoxicity

Many drugs exhibit a selective toxicity to the kidney, including antibiotics such as the sulfonamides. A major route of sulfonamide metabolism is by acetylation of the 4-amino group in the molecule, a pathway that results in pharmacological inactivation. However, an occasional toxic effect of the sulfonamides is crystalluria, a condition caused by precipitation of the less soluble acetylated sulfonamide metabolite in the tubular urine, especially when the urine is acidic.

In addition, the kidney has significant amounts of the mixed-function oxidase system enzymes and prostaglandin endoperoxide synthetase, two enzyme systems that have the potential to metabolically activate innocuous drugs and chemicals to toxic metabolites. Although our knowledge of the kidney metabolism of xenobiotics is not as fully developed as the equivalent system in the liver, it is becoming clearer that the kidney can also activate drugs. For example, paracetamol can be metabolised both by mixed-function oxidation and by co-oxidation in the presence of arachidonic acid and prostaglandin endoperoxide synthetase. Both of these pathways result in the production of toxic metabolites that bind to critical, cellular macromolecules and ultimately result in necrosis of the kidney tissue in a similar fashion to the liver as described above. In addition many urinary bladder carcinogens such as benzidine and many nephrotoxic chlorinated hydrocarbons (including chloroform, carbon tetrachloride and trichloroethylene) require metabolic activation as a necessary prelude to the expression of their nephrotoxicity.

The kidney is apparently susceptible to the toxicity of drugs and chemicals that are metabolised by conjugation with glutathione and subsequent metabolic processing to renal toxins. Toxic compounds in this class include halogenated alkenes

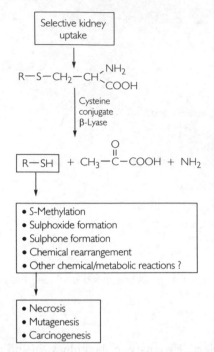

Figure 6.18 Selective kidney uptake and cysteine conjugate β-lyase-dependent bioactivation of xenobiotics. R represents a xenobiotic substrate.

used in the chemical industry, such as hexachlorobutadiene, perchloroethylene and trichloroethylene. As discussed previously, the glutathione adduct of these xenobiotics is metabolised to the corresponding cysteine conjugate which, as an organic anion, is selectively taken up and concentrated in the P_3 segment of the proximal convoluted tubule, coincident with the kidney localisation of the cysteine conjugate β-lyase enzyme, which further metabolises the compound to necrotic, mutagenic and carcinogenic metabolites (Figure 6.18). However, it must be borne in mind that predisposition to the nephrotoxicity of compounds metabolised via this pathway depends on many factors, with the overall balance of activating/deactivating enzymes playing a major role.

Neurotoxicity
The blood–brain barrier is a membrane-based, specialised neuroanatomical structure that normally protects the central nervous system from exposure to blood-borne toxicants, but in the case of drugs and xenobiotics, their relatively high lipid solubility facilitates penetration. Thus xenobiotics have the potential to express neurotoxicity and indeed, it has been estimated that approximately 28% of industrial chemicals are potential neurotoxins. Many neurotoxicants are direct acting, but as with most other tissues, toxicity in the central nervous system may additionally be mediated through metabolites (Table 6.8). Metabolites may be formed at

Table 6.8 Neurotoxins which act through their metabolites

Parent compound	Toxic metabolite
Parathion	Paraoxon
Cocaine	Norcocaine
MPTP	MPP$^+$
Methanol	Formaldehyde
Ethanol	Acetaldehyde
n-Hexane	2,5-Hexanedione

the site of toxicity as the central nervous system expresses most of the enzymes of drug metabolism, albeit at substantially lower levels than the liver, or (less usually) be transported from the liver.

MPTP (1-methyl-4-phenyl-1,2,3,6-tetrahydropyridine, Figure 6.19) is an impurity in a heroin-like 'designer street drug' of abuse (MPPP, a pethidine analogue), whose neurotoxicity first came to light in southern California, where young abusers exhibited symptoms of central nervous system toxicity that were remarkably similar to that of advanced Parkinson's disease. Subsequent intensive research revealed that the site of toxicity of MPTP was the dopaminergic neurones of the substantia nigra, the precise locus of the degenerative aetiology of Parkinson's in the elderly. MPTP is not directly toxic *per se*, but must be metabolised, initially in the astrocyte, by monoamine oxidase B to MPDP$^+$ and subsequent oxidation to MPP$^+$ (Figure 6.19). MPP$^+$ is subsequently excreted from the astrocyte where it is actively taken up into dopaminergic neurones by an active transport system and finally exerts its toxicity by inhibiting mitochondrial NADH dehydrogenase, thereby inhibiting oxidative phosphorylation and ATP production, an early prelude to cell death.

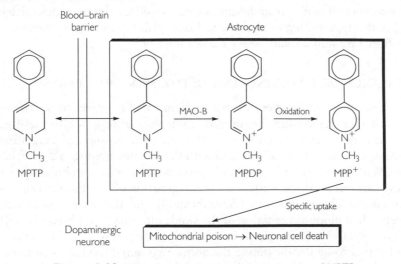

Figure 6.19 Role of metabolism in the neurotoxicity of MPTP.

Table 6.9 Role of glucuronic acid conjugation in the toxicity of xenobiotics in the rabbit and cat

Compound	LD$_{50}$ (mg/kg)	
	Rabbit	Cat
Phenol	250	80
Paracetamol	1200	250

Adapted from Caldwell, J. (1980) In: *Concepts in Drug Metabolism, Part A* (P. Jenner and B. Testa, eds). Marcel Dekker, New York.

6.3.2 Metabolism resulting in decreased toxicity

From the above discussion, it is clear that many phase 1 reactions result in the production of toxic metabolites of xenobiotics. However, this phenomenon must not be considered in isolation as many of the toxic phase 1 metabolites are substrates of phase 2 enzymes, the resultant conjugate, in general, being considerably less toxic than the initial metabolite. It must be clearly understood that metabolism is generally a detoxification reaction for the majority of xenobiotics and that metabolic activation is viewed as the exception to the rule.

For example, paracetamol is activated by the mixed-function oxidase system but, in low doses, the reactive metabolite (Figure 6.16) is conjugated with cellular glutathione and safely excreted as thiol conjugates. This protective influence of the phase 2 enzymes is clearly seen in experimental animals depleted of cellular glutathione by compounds such as diethyl maleate. Such glutathione-depleted animals are then rendered more susceptible to paracetamol hepatotoxicity, whereas the animals are protected against the toxicity of this analgesic by glutathione or N-acetylcysteine (glutathione precursor) supplementation.

Another example of phase 2 metabolism resulting in decreased toxicity is seen in glucuronidation reactions when comparing the LD$_{50}$ values of various compounds in species that have different abilities to form glucuronide conjugates. Whereas the rabbit is competent at glucuronidation, the cat is well known to be defective in this phase 2 pathway, resulting in an increased susceptibility to various compounds, as demonstrated by substantially lower LD$_{50}$ values (Table 6.9).

6.4 BALANCE OF TOXIFYING AND DETOXIFYING PATHWAYS

If a drug can be metabolised either to a toxic metabolite or inactivated by metabolism, what then determines the ultimate toxicological response to the drug? An obvious answer to this question is that there is a balance of activating and deactivating enzymes, as is exemplified with the hepatocarcinogen 2-acetylaminofluorene. With reference to Figure 6.12, two main routes of metabolism exist. The first is cytochrome P450-dependent monooxygenation of the fluorenyl ring system and subsequent glucuronidation (detoxification) and the second is cytochrome P450-dependent monooxygenation of the amide nitrogen and subsequent sulfation of the hydroxylamine (activation). In the first instance, it is thought that different forms of cytochrome P450 catalyse the above two initial oxidation reactions and therefore the relative amounts and activities of these isoforms will determine, in

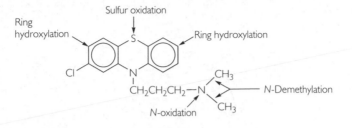

Figure 6.20 Multiple phase I metabolic pathways for chlorpromazine.

part, the ultimate biological response. In addition, Figure 6.12 demonstrates that sulfate esterification of the N-hydroxy metabolite is a key metabolic step in the activation of this compound to a carcinogen. Thus it is clear that the concentration and activity of the cytoplasmic sulfotransferase enzymes are a major determinant of the hepatic toxicity of 2-acetylaminofluorene. Accordingly, species such as the guinea pig, which have low hepatic sulfotransferase activity, are resistant to 2-acetylaminofluorene-induced hepatic cancer.

As shown in Figure 6.20, the phase 1 metabolism of the anti-psychotic/sedative drug chlorpromazine is complex, consisting of ring hydroxylation, N-demethylation, S-oxidation and N-oxidation reactions occurring in the microsomal fraction of the hepatocyte. In fact, the metabolism of this drug is even more complex when the phase 2 glucuronidation and sulfation reactions are taken into account, resulting in the excretion of approximately 20–30 different metabolites in human urine. At present, although the pharmacological and toxicological potencies of these various metabolites have not all been definitively characterised, it is likely that the metabolites have different potencies and the metabolism of this drug is another illustration of the importance of the balance of metabolic pathways in determining the ultimate biological response.

The metabolism of the organic compound bromobenzene serves as another excellent example of the importance of the balance between toxifying and detoxifying enzymes. Bromobenzene is hepatotoxic and in sufficiently high doses may result in the expression of hepatic necrosis in experimental animals fed this compound. Many studies have shown that bromobenzene requires metabolic activation to express its hepatotoxicity, but it must be emphasised that other detoxifying metabolic pathways exist (Figure 6.21). Initially, bromobenzene is metabolised to the key reactive metabolite bromobenzene-3,4-epoxide by the cytochrome P450-dependent mixed-function oxidase system. This reaction is preferentially catalysed by a phenobarbitone-induced form of cytochrome P450 whereas epoxidation of bromobenzene is directed towards the 2,3 position by a polycyclic aromatic hydrocarbon-induced variant of the haemoprotein (CYP1A1). The prevailing balance of these cytochromes P450 is an important determinant of bromobenzene toxicity as the 3,4 epoxide is considerably more toxic to the liver cell than the 2,3 epoxide. Once formed, the 3,4 epoxide may have several different fates (Figure 6.21). The epoxide may be inactivated by diol formation

195

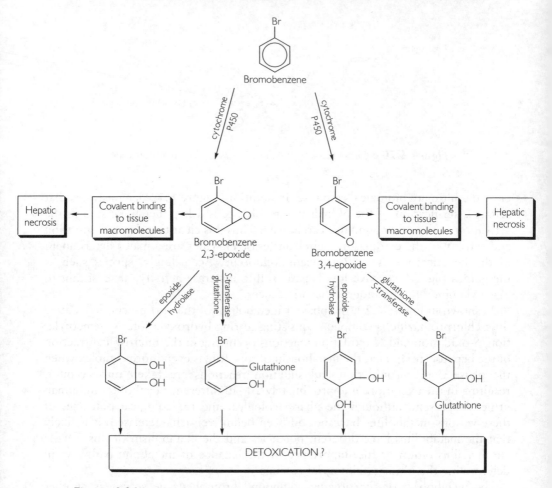

Figure 6.21 Metabolic activation and inactivation of the hepatotoxin, bromobenzene.

(catalysed by the enzyme epoxide hydrolase), glutathione conjugation (catalysed by the glutathione *S*-transferases) or covalently bind to critical tissue macromolecules, the presumed chemico-biological interaction that initiates cellular necrosis. It has also been postulated that the hepatotoxicity of bromobenzene is associated with the cellular depletion of glutathione (as a direct result of metabolism) and hence the attendant potential toxicity associated with substantial changes in cellular glutathione homeostasis. Although the precise mechanism(s) of bromobenzene-induced hepatic toxicity have yet to be elucidated, it should be clear from the above discussion that the balance of the metabolising enzymes and the availability of glutathione is an important determinant of toxicity.

One important feature of the phase 2 reactions is that they are quite frequently capacity-limited by the availability of the endogenous compound required for conjugation with the parent drug or its phase 1 metabolite (Table 6.10).

Table 6.10 Capacities of conjugation reactions

Capacity	Reaction
High	Glucuronidation
Medium	Amino acid conjugation
Low	Sulfation and glutathione conjugation
Variable	Acetylation

Adapted from Caldwell, J. (1980) In: *Concepts in Drug Metabolism, Part A* (P. Jenner and B. Testa, eds), Marcel Dekker, New York.

Table 6.11 Detoxification failure due to saturation of conjugation reactions

Compound	Species	Saturatable reaction	Nature of toxicity
Paracetamol, bromobenzene	Several	Glutathione conjugation	Hepatocellular necrosis
Chloramphenicol	Human neonate	Glucuronidation	Agranulocytosis
Benzoic acid	Cat	Glycine conjugation	Death
Phenol	Cat	Sulfation	Death

Adapted from Caldwell, J. (1980) In: *Concepts in Drug Metabolism, Part A* (P. Jenner and B. Testa, eds), Marcel Dekker, New York.

This capacity-limited phenomenon is readily understood because many of the endogenous conjugating molecules, such as glucuronic acid, sulfate and glutathione, are additionally required for the metabolism and conjugation of endogenous substrates such as steroids and bile acids. Accordingly, when the body is challenged with high doses of drugs, higher than normal levels of conjugating molecules are required for metabolism. If the synthesis of the endogenous conjugating compounds is limited in any way then a predictable result of drug therapy in high doses would be the inability to conjugate the drug in question. In the majority of cases, where phase 2 conjugation reactions result in detoxification, failure to conjugate the drug would then result in an overt expression of drug-induced toxicity (Table 6.11).

A good example of the capacity-limited conjugation of drugs is seen with aspirin excretion in man. As shown in Figure 6.22, aspirin can be conjugated with either the amino acid glycine or with glucuronic acid. At low doses of aspirin, glycine conjugation is the main metabolic pathway. However, on increasing the aspirin dose, the glycine conjugating system becomes readily saturated and conjugation switches to glucuronide formation. At the highest doses of aspirin, the glucuronidation system also becomes saturated, and salicylic acid becomes a major excretory product.

6.5 ASSESSMENT OF HUMAN DRUG METABOLISING ENZYMES IN PHARMACOLOGY AND TOXICOLOGY

Most of the examples described so far in the pharmacological and toxicological aspects of drug metabolism relate to the use of purified animal enzymes or tissue

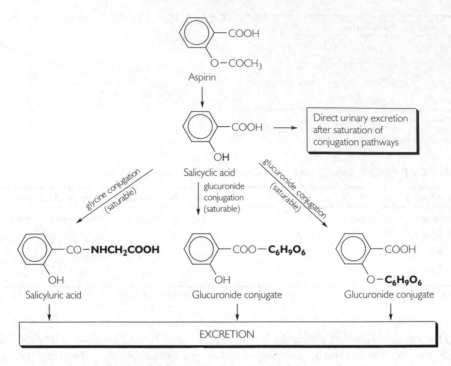

Figure 6.22 Capacity-limited metabolism of aspirin.

preparations. Because of practical and ethical reasons, it is obviously much more difficult to gather the same amount of sophisticated biological information on human drug-metabolising enzymes. However, with the advent of rapid advances in molecular biology and biotechnology, many of the human enzymes have been cloned and expressed in heterologous cell-based systems, thereby allowing a more facile and incisive approach to assessing human activation/deactivation potential for drugs and xenobiotics (Figure 6.23). Although there are many refinements yet to be made and a few pitfalls associated with this type of approach, it offers excellent potential for exciting developments in understanding human enzymology and toxicology. The reader is referred to Section 7.3 for a fuller discussion of the assessment of the methods used to assess drug metabolism in man.

Another area of expanding interest is the need to assess the potential of chemicals to induce human drug-metabolising enzymes. Notwithstanding ethical and practical reasons, this is difficult to do *in vivo* as probe substrates used to assess induction of, say, a particular form of human cytochrome P450 are, at best, only *relatively* specific for a particular form and other forms may contribute. *In vitro* approaches to assessing human metabolism have been extensively used in the form of hepatocyte primary cultures or precision-cut liver slices, but suffer from the disadvantage that fresh and viable human liver is not always readily available and

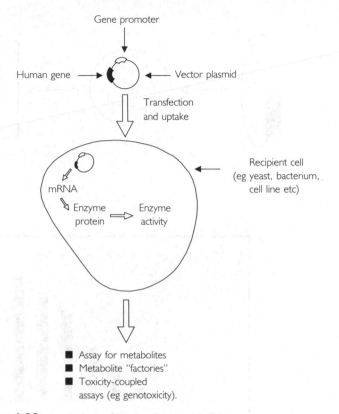

Figure 6.23 Assessment of human drug metabolising enzymes.

that hepatocytes/liver slices rapidly de-differentiate in culture, resulting in the loss of enzymes.

A significant move forward in assessing the ability of drugs and chemicals to induce human liver drug-metabolising enzymes has been the use of promoter/ reporter gene constructs *in vitro*. As shown for CYP3A4 in Figure 6.24, the CYP3A4 promoter (regulatory region) is coupled to a reporter gene whose enzyme activity is readily measured and is a surrogate for transcriptional activation of the CYP3A4 promoter. If cellular receptors and other transcription factors contribute to the induction process, then the system may be refined by co-transfection of the cognate cDNAs (in an expression plasmid) in stable human liver cell lines. Although the system described above for CYP3A4 (and indeed for other enzyme systems) is still an *in vitro* system, it retains dose–response characteristics to inducers and is capable of identifying almost all of the known *in vivo* inducers of CYP3A4.

Another recent development in the characterisation of human drug-metabolising enzymes is the ability to stably incorporate a full length cDNA into the genome of a recipient cell, the latter acting as a reporter of toxicity when the cognate xenobiotic substrate is added to the cell culture system. As shown in Figure 6.25, this approach

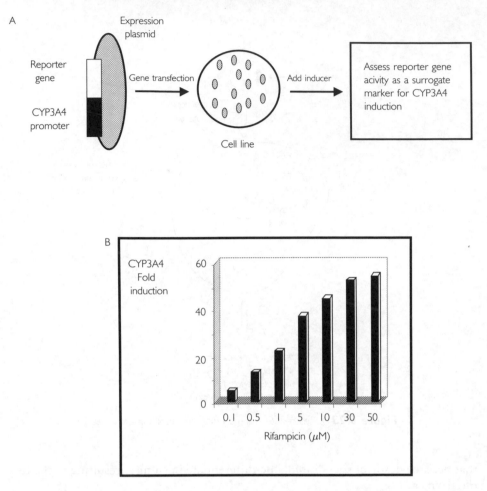

Figure 6.24 Use of promoter/reporter gene constructs to identify and characterise inducers of human CYP3A4. A is a schematic of the reporter gene system and B represents a dose–response curve to rifampicin (a classical inducer of CYP3A4) in this system.

has been taken to compare and contrast the ability of rat and human cysteine conjugate β-lyases to metabolically activate dichlorovinyl cysteine (DCVC), thus providing valuable human data for the risk assessment of these metabolic conjugates to man.

6.6 CONCLUSIONS

The classical viewpoint of drug metabolism being a detoxifying pathway is no longer entirely true. Although many examples are known where metabolism results in decreased pharmacological and toxicological responses, it must be emphasised

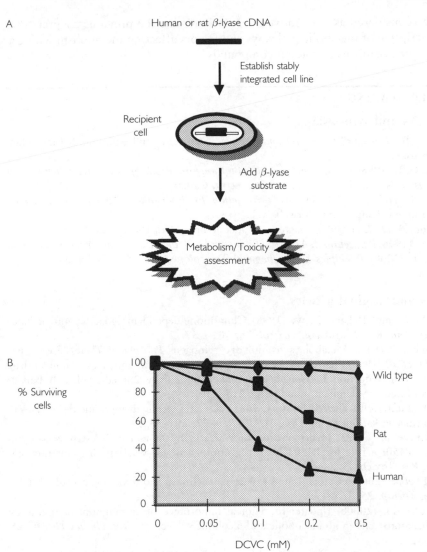

A Human or rat β-lyase cDNA

Establish stably
integrated cell line

Recipient
cell

Add β-lyase
substrate

Metabolism/Toxicity
assessment

B % Surviving cells

Wild type

Rat

Human

DCVC (mM)

Figure 6.25 Stable cell line engineering of cysteine conjugate β-lyase and use in metabolism and toxicity assessment. A is a schematic of the cell system, engineered to have stably incorporated the rat or human cysteine conjugate β-lyase genes. B is comparative dose–response curves for the ability of dichlorovinyl cysteine to produce cell death after metabolism by either rat or human cysteine conjugate β-lyases. The wild type refers to the parental cell (pig kidney LLC PK1 cells) which was unmodified.

that activation reactions have also been amply verified. This chapter has focused on specific examples of activation and inactivation and emphasis has been placed on the critical role played by the balance of the drug-metabolising enzymes in determining the ultimate biological response(s) to the drug. Accordingly, this chapter should be considered as 'integrative', i.e. consolidating the previous chapters that were descriptive of metabolic pathways and factors affecting metabolism with the responses of organisms to foreign compounds.

FURTHER READING

Textbooks and symposia

Ballantyne. B. *et al.* (1999) *General and Applied Toxicology*, 2nd edn, vol. 2. Macmillan, Basingstoke.

Hawkins, D.R. (1988–1996) *A Survey of the Biotransformations of Drugs and Chemicals in Animals*, vols 1–7. Royal Society of Chemistry, Cambridge.

Hodgson, E. and Levi, P.E. (1994) *Introduction to Biochemical Toxicology*, 2nd edn. Appleton and Lange, East Norwalk, CT.

Marquardt. H. *et al.* (1999) *Toxicology*. Academic Press, San Diego, CA.

Prescott, L. (1996) *Paracetamol: A Critical Bibliographic Review*. Taylor and Francis, London.

Timbrell, J. (2000) *Principles of Biochemical Toxicology*, 3rd edn. Taylor and Francis, London.

Reviews and original articles

Anders, M.W. and Dekant, M.W. (1998) Glutathione-dependent bioactivation of halo-alkenes. *Ann. Rev. Pharmacol. Toxicol.* 38, 501–537.

Guengerich, F.P. (1992) Metabolic activation of carcinogens. *Pharmacol. Therap.* 54, 17–61.

Hadidi, H. *et al.* (1999) Pharmacogenetics and toxicological consequences of human drug oxidation and reduction. In: *General and Applied Toxicology*, 2nd edn, vol. 1 (B. Ballantyne *et al.*, eds). Macmillan, London, pp 215–250.

Maret, O. *et al.* (1990) The MPTP story: MAO activates tetrahydropyridine derivatives to toxins causing Parkinsonism. *Drug Metab. Rev.* 22, 291–332.

Rettie, A.E. *et al.* (1992) Hydroxylation of warfarin by human cDNA-expressed cytochrome P450: a role for P4502C9 in the etiology of (*S*)-warfarin-drug interactions. *Chem. Res. Toxicol.* 5, 54–59.

Tanaka, E. *et al.* (2000a) Cytochrome P450 2E1: its clinical and toxicological role. *J. Clin. Pharm. Therap.* 25, 165–175.

Tanaka, E. *et al.* (2000b) Update: the clinical importance of acetaminophen (paracetamol) hepatotoxicity in non-alcoholic and alcoholic subjects. *J. Clin. Pharm. Therap.* 25, 325–332.

Tweats, D.J. and Gatehouse, D.G. (1999) Mutagenicity. In: *General and Applied Toxicology*, 2nd edn, vol. 2 (B. Ballantyne *et al.*, eds). Macmillan, Basingstoke, pp 1017–1078.

7 THE CLINICAL RELEVANCE OF DRUG METABOLISM

LEARNING OBJECTIVES

At the end of this chapter, you should be able to:
- Describe the one- and two-compartment models of pharmacokinetics
- Define drug half-life, volume of distribution, elimination rate constant, clearance (including hepatic clearance) and their inter-relationship
- Define and explain the relevance of first- and zero-order kinetics
- Describe the relevance of the absorption compartment
- Describe, using examples, the methods used to study drug metabolism in man and discuss the advantages, disadvantages and relevance of each method
- Discuss *in vitro/in vivo* correlations in drug metabolism

7.1 INTRODUCTION

The ultimate aim for most studies in drug metabolism, even those initially using animal models, is to ascertain what happens in man with a view to relating this to the action of the drug or its metabolite(s). Drug metabolism in man is more difficult to study than in animals, due to the practical and ethical constraints on experimentation. There is only limited ethical access to tissue samples and it is difficult to find a reasonably homogeneous group of subjects on which to perform the studies. Different approaches to the study of drug metabolism have to be adopted in man as routine procedures – the most usual of which is the measurement of drug concentrations in blood plasma over an extended time period. Other biological fluids (such as urine or saliva) may also be used where appropriate and validated. More recently the use of cultured or isolated cells has become more widespread. These methods are discussed later.

When considering the action of a drug (or, indeed, its active, perhaps toxic, metabolite), the two most important parameters are its intensity and duration of action. These are related directly to the concentration of drug at its site of action and the time during which the effective concentration of drug remains there. It is often difficult to assess the concentration of a drug at its actual site of action but, fortunately, the concentration of drug in the blood plasma is most often a good measure of this. Measurement of plasma concentrations of drugs and how these change is, therefore, an important exercise in determining drug action. One of the main contributors to the change in active drug concentration in plasma is the metabolism of the drug. Remember, however, that metabolism may create or destroy an active drug molecule and, thus, can increase or decrease its action (see Chapter 6). The theoretical and mathematical interpretation of tissue drug concentration data is termed *pharmacokinetics*.

Pharmacokinetics is particularly important from a clinical view because of the relationship between the intensity and duration of action of a drug, the concentration of drug present at the active site and how long an effective concentration is found there, respectively. The ability to calculate the concentration of drug in the plasma at a particular time point can be vital in assessing the dose and frequency of dosing of a drug of low therapeutic index, e.g. anticoagulants, cardiac glycosides or anti-cancer drugs. The ability to correlate *in vivo* pharmacokinetic and metabolic data with *in vitro* metabolic data is also important. Does increased drug metabolism have any effect on clearance of drugs from the body? This question is examined in detail later.

Pharmacokinetics will be considered mainly from a physiological point of view but mathematical equations will be given where they assist in the understanding of the principles (no derivations of equations will be given; these can be found in any standard pharmacokinetics textbook and are of little relevance here). The special relevance of the hepatic drug-metabolising capacity to pharmacokinetics will be highlighted. The methods of obtaining clinical data related to drug metabolism will also be discussed and the increasingly important correlation of *in vivo* and *in vitro* data considered. Finally, specific examples of the clinical relevance of drug metabolism will be given, with a discussion of the wider implications of various factors affecting pharmacokinetic parameters, such as induction/inhibition, disease states and dietary control.

7.2 PHARMACOKINETICS

Pharmacokinetics (literally, the movement of drugs) is the study of the uptake, distribution and clearance (by excretion and/or metabolism) of drugs with respect to time. In practice this means measuring the concentration of drug in various tissues and body fluids over a period of time and fitting them to a mathematical model. The processes involved in the determination of pharmacokinetic patterns are illustrated in Figure 7.1. In order to interpret the pharmacokinetic data, it is necessary to set up certain models of the body so that the mathematical equations describing the movement of the drugs can be formulated. First we will briefly describe two simple, well-used models to illustrate how this may be done and then describe some of the newer physiologically based pharmacokinetic models being developed.

7.2.1 The one-compartment model

It can be appreciated from Figure 7.1 that the movement of drug between different compartments of the body (blood, adipose tissue, gut, liver, etc.) is a complex, dynamic process and not readily amenable to simple, direct analysis. It is therefore assumed, as a first approximation in this model, that all body compartments are in rapid equilibrium with a central compartment (normally equated with the blood), and that the concentration of drug is constant throughout, i.e. the body is considered as a single compartment through which the drug equilibrates instantaneously. The actual correlation of pharmacokinetic compartments with real anatomical tissues or organs in this model is not considered (as the body is defined

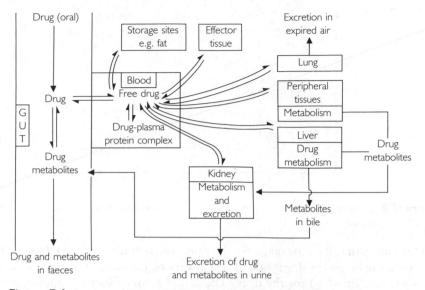

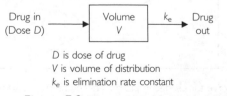

Figure 7.1 Processes involved in the determination of pharmacokinetic parameters.

as one compartment) and this should be borne in mind during these discussions. Using this approximation, a pharmacokinetic model can be constructed as in Figure 7.2. This is the *one-compartment model*.

It is assumed that the drug is injected directly into this compartment (e.g. intravenous injection) and distributes itself instantaneously through the compartment. Thus the concentration of drug at time zero (C_0) can be calculated or conversely, if C_0 is known, V can be calculated:

$$C_0 = D/V \quad \text{or} \quad V = D/C_0 \tag{7.1}$$

where
  V is the volume of distribution
  D is the dose of drug.

Clearance of the drug from the compartment then takes place at a rate determined by the elimination rate constant (k_e). For most drugs this clearance is directly related to the concentration of drug, i.e. a plot of log drug concentration versus time yields a straight line (referred to as first-order kinetics) (Figure 7.3).

Drug in (Dose D) → Volume V → k_e → Drug out

D is dose of drug
V is volume of distribution
k_e is elimination rate constant

Figure 7.2 The one-compartment model.

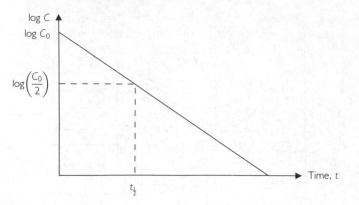

Figure 7.3 Theoretical curve for change in plasma drug concentration in the one-compartment model.

This means that the time taken for the drug concentration to halve (wherever on the curve the original value is taken) will always be the same. This time is referred to as the half-life ($t_{1/2}$) for the drug. The actual form of such a semi-log plot for real data is usually similar to that shown in Figure 7.4. The deviation of the actual and theoretical curves at the start is due to distribution of the drug taking a finite time (not instantaneous as the model demands); therefore the sampled (plasma) compartment has a higher concentration of drug than the body as a whole.

Various parameters can be measured or calculated for a first-order, one-compartment model:

$$V = \text{volume of distribution}$$
$$C_0 = \text{concentration of drug at time 0}$$
$$C_t = \text{concentration of drug at various times}$$
$$t_{1/2} = \text{half-life of elimination}$$
$$k_e = \text{elimination rate constant}$$
$$D = \text{dose of drug given.}$$

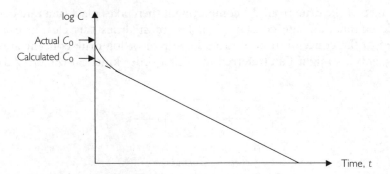

Figure 7.4 Experimental curve for change in plasma concentration of a drug approximating to the one-compartment model.

The elimination rate constant (k_e) is defined as the rate of change of drug concentration at unit initial drug concentration (or mathematically as below):

$$dC/dT = -k_e C_0 \qquad (7.2)$$

Using this equation and measurements of plasma drug concentrations at various times, the elimination rate constant can be calculated. The elimination rate constant is a composite figure encompassing all methods of elimination (excretion in urine, faeces, expired air, sweat, etc., biotransformation and sequestration in tissues not sampled). It is almost impossible to separate it into its components and this is important when discussing the correlations between *in vivo* and *in vitro* measures of drug metabolism (see Section 7.4).

If the equation above is expressed in another form:

$$\log C = \log C_0 - k_e t \log e \qquad (7.3)$$

then a relationship between k_e and $t_{1/2}$ can be seen:

$$\log[C/C_0] = -k_e t \log e \qquad (7.4)$$

where $e = $ the exponential function (log $e = 0.434$).
At $t_{1/2}$, $C = C_0/2$. Thus $\log\frac{1}{2} = -0.301 = -0.434 k_e t$ and

$$k_e = \frac{0.693}{t_{1/2}}. \qquad (7.5)$$

So the elimination rate constant is inversely proportional to the half-life of the drug. This is quite logical, as the faster the clearance of the drug (greater k_e) the faster one-half of the drug will be cleared and therefore the shorter the half-life.

So, overall, we can see that the rate at which a drug is cleared from the body is dependent on a complex elimination rate constant, the dose of drug and the body volume through which the drug is distributed:

$$dC/dT = k_e D/V. \qquad (7.6)$$

The volume of distribution of a drug is also a complex 'constant'. In physiological terms it is sometimes difficult to equate calculated volumes of distribution with actual body compartments. The drug may only enter the blood plasma and have a small volume of distribution (say 3 L), or it may enter the extracellular fluid or even permeate all cells (total body water), thus giving a large volume of distribution (say 50 L). More often, the calculated volume of distribution lies somewhere in between. In certain circumstances a volume of distribution greater than the body volume can be obtained. This is a function of the way in which volume of distribution is calculated from a measurement of plasma concentration of drug. The plasma concentration of drug may be very low due to sequestration of drug in, say, adipose tissue; therefore the volume of distribution according to (7.1) will seem to be very large, sometimes measured in hundreds of litres, whereas in reality it is small (only distributed in adipose tissue).

The simple model of the body as a single compartment appears to be reasonably accurate for many drugs and can yield some useful information on the movement, intensity and duration of action of drugs within the body and can lead to the calculation of some important parameters of drug action (e.g. volume of distribution, half-life and elimination rate constant). The problems with the interpretation of these parameters should, however, be remembered.

7.2.2 The two-compartment model

The one-compartment model discussed above assumes that elimination can occur from every compartment of the body and that the drug can enter all areas of the body equally easily, but a glance at Figure 7.1 shows that this may not always be valid: many peripheral tissues cannot excrete directly and excretion takes place mainly from the blood (via urine or faeces). A refinement can be added to the one-compartment model to account for this in the form of an outer, non-excreting compartment (Figure 7.5). This is called the *two-compartment model*, where the two compartments are kinetically distinguishable.

Such a model is more complex to analyse and mathematically gives a plot of log drug concentration in the central compartment versus time as shown in Figure 7.6. There are two distinct slopes, the first (steeper) slope being primarily related to distribution of drug from the central to the peripheral compartment, and the second (shallower) slope to the elimination of drug from the central compartment. The second half-life ($t_{1/2}$) is the true half-life of elimination as defined earlier. This theoretical slope more closely follows the actual experimental plots found for some drugs and thus can be considered a more realistic model.

The central compartment in this model is generally equated with the blood plasma and other non-fatty highly perfused tissues and the peripheral compartment with other tissues (Table 7.1). Which of the tissues are included in the central and which in the peripheral compartment depends on the drug in question.

As can be imagined, mathematical analysis of a two-compartment model is more complex than that of a one-compartment model and, although all parameters calculated from the one-compartment model can also be calculated from this

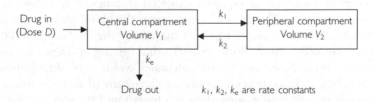

Figure 7.5 The two-compartment model.

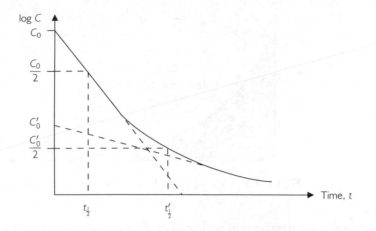

Figure 7.6 Theoretical curve for the change in plasma drug concentration in the two-compartment model.

Description of group	Tissues
Plasma	Plasma
Highly perfused non-fat	Blood cells
	Heart
	Lung
	Liver
	Kidney
	Glands
Poorly perfused non-fat	Muscle
	Skin
Fatty tissues	Adipose tissue
	Bone marrow
Negligible perfusion	Bone
	Teeth
	Cartilage
	Hair

Table 7.1 Tissue groupings for pharmacokinetic assessment

model, one further parameter is necessary to understand the analysis, i.e. the area under the concentration–time curves (AUC). This is exactly what its name suggests, the area under the curve when plasma drug concentration is plotted against time (Figure 7.7).

The area under the curve is a measure of the total body load of drug (i.e. its bioavailability) and is therefore an indirect indication of the therapeutic value of the drug. Provided clearance of the drug remains constant, changes in AUC relate to changes in bioavailability of the drug (for instance, by giving the drug by different routes). The AUC can be measured experimentally and used to calculate the clearance of drug from the body as below. Clearance is defined as the volume of

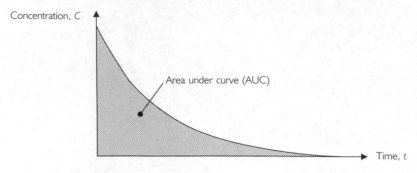

Figure 7.7 The area under the concentration–time curve.

the central compartment that is cleared of drug in unit time, and thus is a measure of the efficiency with which a drug is eliminated from the body via all routes.

$$\text{Clearance} = D/\text{AUC} \tag{7.7}$$

where D is the dose of drug given.

Clearance can also be expressed in terms of the elimination rate constant:

$$\text{Clearance} = k_e v_1 \tag{7.8}$$

where k_e is the elimination rate constant and v_1 is the volume of the central compartment.

Clearance is a very important concept in pharmacokinetics and therapeutics, as we will see later.

A number of problems are inherent in the two-compartment model. One problem is the fact that the concentration of drug in the central compartment is no longer related solely to drug elimination but also to movement of drug between the central and peripheral compartments. It depends on the relative rate constants (k_1, k_2 and k_e) whether movement of drug or elimination is the most important and, thus, analysis of changes in drug concentration becomes more complex. A second problem is more pharmacological and relates to the position of the receptor for the drug. The intensity of action of the drug is related to the concentration of drug at its receptor. Thus, analysis of drug concentrations in both compartments is strictly necessary to evaluate the relevance of pharmacokinetic data to clinical use of the drug using a two-compartment model. The difficulty of assigning anatomical regions to the various compartments makes this more difficult.

7.2.3 Kinetic order of reaction

One final theoretical consideration to be discussed is the kinetic order of reaction. All of the theory so far discussed assumes that the elimination of drug is directly related to its concentration (i.e. the elimination is first order). This is the normal situation for a chemical reaction based on the law of mass action. If, however,

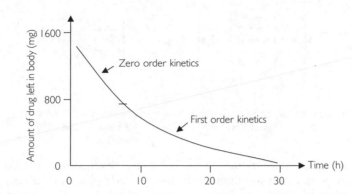

Figure 7.8 Clearance of acetylsalicylic acid in man. (Taken from Levy, G. (1965) *J. Pharm. Sci.* **54**, 959.)

the processes of elimination are saturated (normally at high drug concentrations where one of the other components of the reaction becomes rate-limiting, such as a co-factor), elimination rate is independent of drug concentration (i.e. zero-order kinetics) and drug is being cleared as fast as possible. In this case a plot of drug concentration versus time is linear. This can be seen very well with higher doses of aspirin (Figure 7.8). At first, acetylsalicylate concentration falls linearly with time until sub-saturation is reached, when first-order kinetics reappear. One drug that is nearly always cleared by zero-order kinetics is ethanol (alcohol) where the co-factor, NAD^+, is the rate-limiting factor and not the ethanol.

In exceptional circumstances, involving two or more substances in metabolism or excretion, multi-order kinetics can be seen but such instances are rare.

7.2.4 Pharmacokinetics in the clinical situation

In clinical practice it is unusual to give a drug as a single intravenous dose. It is more usual to give multiple doses by a method other than intravenous injection. Consideration of multiple drug dosing and other forms of administration is therefore in order.

Let us first examine a drug administered in a way that does not give direct entry into the central compartment (e.g. oral administration) and which therefore involves absorption of the drug. In these cases the drug first enters another compartment, the absorption compartment. This is an extension of the one- or two-compartment model outlined above (Figure 7.9). The drug is subsequently distributed to the central compartment (and, in the case of the two-compartment model, to the peripheral compartment) and excreted. It can be seen that absorption could still be proceeding as distribution and elimination starts, and this gives the log dose–response curves as shown in Figure 7.10(a) for the one-compartment and 7.10(b) for the two-compartment model. For the one-compartment model both the absorption rate constant (k_a) and the elimination rate constant (k_e) can be calculated by extrapolation of the respective curves and by using the equations given

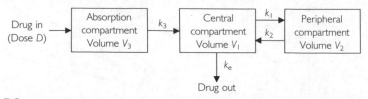

Figure 7.9 Modification of one- and two-compartment models to include the absorption compartment. (Taken from Levy, G. (1965) *J. Pharm. Sci.* **54**, 959.)

earlier. In the two-compartment model, however, absorption, distribution and elimination are proceeding simultaneously and the early phase of the curve cannot be analysed satisfactorily. Further complications arise in oral dosing as the rate of dissolution of the drug must also be taken into account. Pharmacokinetic data from orally administered drugs are, therefore, sometimes very difficult to interpret.

Most drugs are administered for an extended period of time and it is of great interest to the clinician to know what dose and at what dosage interval to give a drug in order to achieve an effective drug concentration at its site of action. A consideration of the kinetics of multiple dosing is thus of interest.

The effect of multiple dosing depends on the relationship between the half-life of the drug and the frequency of dosing. If the dosing interval is much longer than the half-life then the dose will be effectively cleared before the next is given and each dose can be considered as entirely separate. If, however, the dosage interval is about

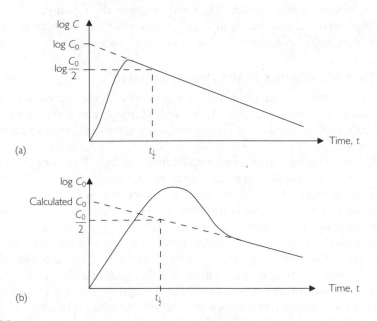

Figure 7.10 Theoretical curve for change in plasma drug concentration in the modified (a) one- and (b) two-compartment models.

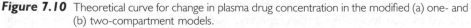

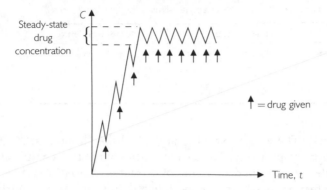

Figure 7.11 Theoretical curve for change in plasma drug concentration on multiple dosing.

$t_{1/2}$ or less, then accumulation of drug occurs until a steady-state concentration is reached (Figure 7.11). The steady-state concentration of drug is dependent on the dose of drug given, the fraction of drug absorbed, the half-life of the drug, the volume of distribution and the dose interval:

$$C = \frac{1.44t_{1/2}FD}{Vi} \qquad (7.9)$$

where C is the steady state concentration, $t_{1/2}$ is the half-life, F is the fraction of drug absorbed, D is the dose of drug, V is the volume of distribution and i is the dose interval.

Factors affecting drug half-life, absorption and volume of distribution thus affect the steady state concentration of drug during multiple dosing.

7.2.5 Hepatic drug clearance

One of the major methods of removing drug from the central compartment is the hepatic drug metabolism, i.e. removal by conversion to a metabolite. The ability of the liver to remove drug from the blood is related to only two variables, i.e. the intrinsic hepatic clearance (Cl_{int}) and the hepatic blood flow (B):

$$\text{Hepatic clearance} = B[Cl_{int}/(B + Cl_{int})] = BR_e \qquad (7.10)$$

Intrinsic clearance is the maximum ability of the liver to extract drug in the absence of blood flow restrictions. The term $[Cl_{int}/(B + Cl_{int})]$ in (7.10) is referred to as the extraction ratio (R_e).

When intrinsic clearance (Cl_{int}) is very much greater than hepatic blood flow then the extraction ratio approaches 1.0 and hepatic clearance is dependent only on blood flow, i.e. the liver extracts all of the drug presented to it. Thus the more blood passing through the liver the more drug will be extracted. On the other hand, if Cl_{int} is very much less than blood flow, then hepatic clearance is dependent only on Cl_{int}, i.e. the liver extracts as much drug as it can from whatever blood

Table 7.2 Comparison of flow- and metabolism-limited hepatic clearance

	Flow-limited	**Metabolism-limited**
Clearance related to	Blood flow	Intrinsic clearance
Extraction ratio	>0.8	<0.2
Examples	Lignocaine, propranolol	Antipyrine

flow is presented. These two extremes are called flow-limited and metabolism-limited extraction, respectively. The characteristics of the two conditions are summarised in Table 7.2. Intermediate values of extraction ratio (0.2–0.8) give hepatic clearance rates that are dependent on both blood flow and hepatic intrinsic clearance to varying extents. It is clear from this that hepatic clearance of drugs may not only be related to the ability of the liver to metabolise drugs but may also be dependent on factors affecting the hepatic blood flow, such as changes in cardiac output and redistribution of blood flow (e.g. during exercise or stress).

7.2.6 Physiologically based pharmacokinetics

Recent attempts to more closely mimic the actual movement of drugs around the body using physiologically based parameters has met with some success. Models based on process control engineering, where a physical or chemical manufacturing process is modelled by analysing each step in the process and giving it realistic parameters, have been used to describe and calculate pharmacokinetic parameters in animals and man. The STELLA software has been used in this way to build up a reasonable picture of how drugs might move around the body. This gives the ability to estimate the likely concentration of drugs or metabolites in various compartments of the body.

7.2.7 Pharmacokinetics: a summary

The first part of this chapter gives a very brief overview of pharmacokinetics as it relates to drug metabolism. It is not designed as a formal introduction to the subject as a whole but should indicate the physiological correlation of the pharmacokinetic parameters and the relevance of pharmacokinetic analysis to clinical practice. The usefulness of this approach must, however, be tempered by the inability of a purely mathematical analysis to completely mimic the actual behaviour of the organism, due to the complexity of the processes under study. The newer physiologically based analyses may go some way towards counteracting these problems in interpretation.

7.3 METHODS FOR STUDYING DRUG METABOLISM IN MAN

As noted above, one of the major aims of research in drug metabolism is to allow the description of the metabolism of compounds in man, as the ability to metabolise a particular drug may be of prime importance in determining the efficacy,

Methods	Substrates used	**Table 7.3** Methods of assessing drug metabolism in man
In vivo clearance	Antipyrine Phenacetin Caffeine Theophylline Paracetamol Debrisoquine Sparteine Sulfadimidine Mephobarbital Diazepam Mephenytoin Codeine Isoniazid Warfarin	
Breath analysis	Aminopyrine Antipyrine Caffeine Diazepam Erythromycin	
In vitro methods	Various	
Non-invasive methods Plasma bilirubin Urinary 6β-hydroxycortisol		

duration of action and toxicity of the drug. It is of importance to be able to assess the ability of patients to metabolise drugs, especially if the drug has a low therapeutic index and needs to be present in the body at a level close to the toxic threshold (e.g. warfarin, cardiac glycosides and many anti-cancer drugs). Many methods have been developed to try and measure drug-metabolising capacity in man and, in this section, a number of these methods will be outlined and the advantages and disadvantages of the methods briefly discussed together with the problems of interpreting the results obtained. The methods are listed in Table 7.3.

7.3.1 *In vivo* clearance

In vivo clearance is one of the major methods for studying drug metabolism in man and relies on the ability to assay the drug concentration in various body fluids such as blood, urine or saliva. The mathematical theories underlying the measurement of *in vivo* clearance have been discussed above, and study of the models reveals a number of criteria that must be fulfilled before clearance can be equated to drug metabolism. These are:

1 The drug must be rapidly and reproducibly absorbed (preferably 100% absorbed).
2 The drug should be distributed throughout total body water (i.e. equivalent to a one-compartment model).
3 The drug should not bind to tissue or plasma protein (only free drug is metabolised, excreted, etc.).

4 The drug should only be metabolised by the liver with a low extraction ratio (i.e. metabolism is not flow-limited).
5 The drug should have negligible renal clearance (i.e. hepatic clearance is the predominant method of clearance).

If all of these criteria are met then drug clearance serves as a meaningful measure of drug metabolism that is not influenced by hepatic blood flow. If urinary excretion of drug and metabolite is measured then, in addition, the drug and metabolite must be excreted in the urine at the same rate and other excretion pathways should be negligible.

The first model drug that came nearest to this ideal was antipyrine where the drug's half-life and clearance both give a good estimate of hepatic metabolism (indicating one-compartment kinetics).

Antipyrine has a number of other advantages:

1 It is easily measured in body fluids after a dose that is pharmacologically inactive.
2 Salivary pharmacokinetics are similar to plasma pharmacokinetics, therefore saliva can be sampled instead of the more painful and potentially damaging venepuncture.

The disadvantages of antipyrine are relatively minor but should be considered. Antipyrine clearance does not always correlate well with metabolism (clearance) of other drugs and therefore is a poor marker for certain drug-metabolising enzyme activities. This is due to the existence of multiple forms of drug-metabolising enzymes in the human liver. The forms of cytochrome P450 metabolising antipyrine in man are well characterised and, thus, a direct correlation between antipyrine clearance and the activity of specific forms of cytochrome P450 can be made. Antipyrine is metabolised to at least three metabolites, and the kinetics of clearance, although appearing simple, are in fact quite complex:

$$\text{Clearance (total)} = \text{Clearance (a)} + \text{Clearance (b)}$$
$$+ \text{Clearance (c)} + \text{Clearance (rest)}$$

where (a) = metabolite a, (b) = metabolite b, (c) = metabolite c, and (rest) = unchanged drug plus non-identified metabolites.

Total clearance is a complex term, including clearance of all metabolites and unchanged drug: a change in one or more of these parameters leads to a change in total clearance, and opposite changes in two parameters can give no apparent change in total clearance, thus masking the effects. Antipyrine is also an inducer of hepatic drug-metabolising enzymes and therefore repeated tests with the drug should be avoided to prevent misleading results being obtained. Although a very old probe drug, antipyrine is still extensively used in pharmacokinetic studies.

Other model substrates have also been employed as markers of hepatic drug metabolism (see Table 7.3). Of these, phenacetin, caffeine and theophylline are thought to be metabolised by CYP1A2 and thus act as markers of a different form than antipyrine. Theophylline is, perhaps, the best of these, as phenacetin undergoes significant metabolism in the gut wall to the O-de-ethylated product, paracetamol. Caffeine has been more recently introduced but suffers the same drawback as theophylline – abstinence from caffeine-containing beverages (coffee, tea, cola) is necessary during the test period. Probes for CYP2D6 activity are also being used, e.g. debrisoquine and sparteine. Here the metabolite ratio in the urine is used as a measure of metabolism.

Mephenytoin metabolism has been correlated to the existence of CYP2C9 and this may also be correlated to the ability to metabolise mephobarbital and, possibly, diazepam. CYP3A4 is quantitatively the most important form in man and the metabolism of a number of probe drugs such as erythromycin has been reported to correlate to activity of this form. The 6β-hydroxylation of testosterone is also considered as a good indication of the activity of CYP3A4.

For phase 2 metabolism, paracetamol has been suggested as a probe for UDP-glucuronosyltransferase activity as has the appearance of codeine-6-glucuronide in the urine. The assessment of acetylator phenotype is more advanced with a number of test drugs being used. Caffeine, isoniazid and sulfadimidine have all been used to measure N-acetylation by urinary metabolic ratio techniques. Isoniazid N-acetylation can also be determined by saliva analysis.

A number of substrates can be used in the study of drug clearance, many of which are good indicators of hepatic drug metabolism. Critical use of this technique can yield useful information regarding the functioning of the liver in man. A further discussion of the relevance of drug clearance to hepatic drug metabolism can be found in Section 7.2.5.

7.3.2 Breath analysis

This method relies on the hepatic breakdown of certain drugs via demethylation to yield carbon dioxide (CO_2) which is excreted via the lungs. Appropriate radio-labelling (with ^{14}C) of the substrate leads to $^{14}CO_2$ being excreted, which can be collected and measured (Figure 7.12). The example given is aminopyrine but

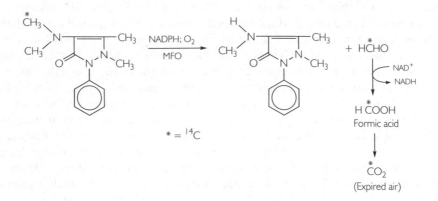

Figure 7.12 The metabolism of ^{14}C-aminopyrine showing release of $^{14}CO_2$ in expired air.

caffeine, antipyrine, diazepam and erythromycin have also been used. The drugs are predominantly metabolised by the hepatic mixed-function oxidase system by N-demethylation and, thus, the CO_2 breath test can be used as an indicator of the functioning of this enzyme system. Indeed the correlation between $^{14}CO_2$ excretion and *in vivo* clearance rate for aminopyrine is good, indicating the relevance of this method. The different substrates also allow assay of different forms of cytochrome P450, e.g. CYP1A2 with caffeine. The disadvantages of this method are that it is assumed that formation of formaldehyde (i.e. drug demethylation) is the rate-limiting step in the production of carbon dioxide (i.e. oxidation of formaldehyde to carbon dioxide is much more rapid than formaldehyde production); this has not been conclusively proved. The patient is also subjected to radioactivity, which is not an ideal situation; a breath test using ^{13}C (a stable non-radioactive form of carbon) is also used which circumvents this objection.

7.3.3 *In vitro* methods

It is clear that if one wishes to investigate drug metabolism in a particular tissue then the best way is to obtain a sample of that tissue and assay the activity directly. If the liver is to be examined, surgical removal of part (or all) of the liver and subjecting it to various tests of drug metabolising ability is the ideal way of gaining information on hepatic drug metabolism. This is the method most commonly employed in animal experiments and is undeniably the most logical. A number of things have to be considered, however, before such studies are initiated in man:

1 ethical considerations
2 sampling procedures
3 assay methods.

Is it ethically acceptable to take a liver sample from a healthy volunteer considering the risks involved in such a procedure? The widely held view is that it is not acceptable, and therefore most human liver material is, to some extent, pathological. It is only acceptable to obtain human liver biopsy material if it is suspected that something is wrong with the liver and no other less stressful method of diagnosis is available. This, of course, means that one is generally dealing with more or less diseased tissue, which makes interpretation of data and extrapolation to the normal human situation difficult. The only time when 'normal' liver may become available is from individuals who have died of a non-liver-related cause, (e.g. during kidney or heart transplant operations (from the donor)). This procedure raises its own ethical problems of consent to removal of organs for medical research – a topic that is very relevant but not within the scope of this book.

From the practical point of view, even if a sample of liver tissue is available it may not be suitable for assay of drug metabolising ability. Samples of liver tissue can be obtained from living patients by percutaneous needle biopsy or wedge biopsy during abdominal surgery. These methods produce fresh tissue directly from the body and are thus subject to minimum disturbance, but only small quantities (milligrams) of tissue can be taken. The size of the sample means that few tests can be performed per patient and also the relevance of the sample is suspect due to the

Table 7.4 Comparison of the methods of liver sampling

Source	Amount	Ethical availability	Reliability	Background knowledge
Needle biopsy	Small	Good[a]	Fair	Good
Wedge biopsy	Small	Good[a]	Fair	Good
Post-mortem	Large	Good	Poor	Fair
Transplant	Large	Poor–fair	Good	Poor

[a] In cases of suspected liver disease; poor in other cases.

known heterogeneity of the liver (differences in drug metabolism between the centrilobular and peripheral areas of the liver). A further complication is the risk involved in obtaining the sample, e.g. infection and internal bleeding from needle biopsy and the inherent risks of major abdominal surgery in taking a wedge biopsy. Larger samples of liver can be obtained following death, e.g. at post mortem. This method has the disadvantage that the liver starts degenerating from the moment of death even if stored cold and, thus, unless obtained relatively soon after death, the liver enzymes may not represent those found during life. Indeed a limit of 2–4 hours after death is put on the liver if it is to be of any use in the study of drug metabolism. As few post mortem examinations are carried out this soon after death, this possible source of liver material is severely limited. One possibility that has been exploited is to remove the liver from clinically dead kidney donors during kidney transplant. From a practical viewpoint this is an excellent method as the liver is virtually normal and functional and so is almost the equivalent of a large biopsy sample. The ethical considerations of this approach are, however, questionable and have been discussed above. One disadvantage of transplant material is the often inadequate background knowledge of the donor (smoking and drinking habits, previous drug use, etc.) which might affect drug-metabolising capacity. A summary of the various sources of human liver material is given in Table 7.4.

Having obtained a sample of liver one has to decide the best preparation to use to assess drug-metabolising capacity. This area has been the focus of intense debate and research over the recent past – how should the scarce human material be collected, stored, distributed and used? Again, these debates are outside the scope of this book but a description of some of the methods developed is appropriate. A list of possible preparations is given in Table 7.5. The range of choice is between a fully physiological preparation (e.g. a whole perfused liver) or a strictly biochemical preparation (e.g. cellular sub-fractions such as microsomes) or

Table 7.5 Liver preparations

Whole liver (perfused)
Liver slices
Liver cubes
Isolated liver cells
Liver homogenate
Isolated liver cell sub-fractions (e.g. microsomes)

Table 7.6 Comparison of liver preparations in assessing drug metabolism

Method	Degree of difficulty	*In vivo* relevance	Reproducibility
Perfused liver	High	Good	Poor
Liver slices	Moderate	Fair	Fair
Liver cubes	Moderate	Fair	Fair
Liver cells	Moderate	Fair	Fair
Subcellular fractions	Low	Fair–poor	Good

a compromise situation (liver slices, cubes and cells). The physiological preparation can only be used if the intact liver is available; it is difficult to set up and keep running. It does, however, give the nearest approximation to the *in vivo* situation. The preparation of subcellular fractions, mainly microsomes derived from the endoplasmic reticulum, is the easiest method but suffers from its non-physiological nature – there is no cellular metabolism, no membrane transport and no endogenous co-factor production. An attempt to reach a mid-point between physiological complexity and biochemical ease has been the use of liver slices and isolated cells. Slices have the physiological cell–cell contact needed for liver function but are somewhat unsatisfactory due to problems of substrate and nutrient access to the centre of the preparation. Isolated liver cells are regarded as the best compromise as they can be kept in culture for extended periods of time without losing their differentiated functions and can be stored frozen and thawed as required for experimentation. The cells isolated from one human liver would be enough for many thousands of assays. Indeed, commercial companies and research organizations now obtain human livers, make and store (deep frozen) liver slices and isolated hepatocytes for use in research and drug testing. The methodology has advanced so far that cells/slices can be provided either embedded in a matrix preserve enzyme activity or pre-attached to cell culture dishes. These liver can be prescreened for drug metabolism characteristics (e.g. total clearance) groups of samples of known activity make up set out for experimentation.

No method of using the liver material obtained is, however, ideal and it depends on the nature of the problem whether a more physiological or biochemical up is required. If changes in enzyme content are under investigation then subfractions may be more appropriate, whereas if hepatotoxicity is being studied whole liver perfusion may lead to the required results. A summary of the ranges and disadvantages of the various methods is given in Table 7.6

In vitro assay of drug-metabolising capacity is the most direct method the techniques employed are relevant to the problem under study ethics are not contravened.

7.3.1 Non-invasive methods

These methods not requiring the administration of a drug are referred invasive. They rely on changes in endogenous metabolism to giv changes in drug metabolism. This is not unreasonable, as much of drug metabolism is related to endogenous compound metabolism, e.g. steroid metabolism is predominantly performed by mixed-function oxidase-like enzymes, neurotransmitters are metabolised by enzymes that also metabolise drugs and glucuronidation is related to glucose metabolism (see Chapter 1 for discussion of the inter-relationship between endogenous and xenobiotic metabolism). The non-invasive techniques that have been used are measurement of plasma gamma-glutamyltransferase (GGT), plasma bilirubin, urinary 6β-hydroxycortisol and urinary D-glucaric acid. Most of these methods, however, are now considered unreliable and do not correlate well with drug metabolism as assayed using the probes described earlier. Only plasma bilirubin levels and the excretion of 6β-hydroxycortisol are still employed to any great extent and then only for specific purposes.

7.3.4.1 Plasma bilirubin

Bilirubin is removed from plasma by conjugation to glucuronic acid in the liver and subsequent excretion. As many drugs also rely on glucuronide conjugation for their excretion, it was thought possible that plasma bilirubin levels could be used as a measure of hepatic glucuronidation (e.g. patients with a genetically low hepatic UDP-glucuronosyltransferase activity – Gilbert's disease – have raised plasma levels of unconjugated bilirubin). No direct comparisons between plasma levels of bilirubin and conjugation of drugs (e.g. chloramphenicol, morphine and oxazepam, which are cleared mainly via glucuronidation in the liver) has been performed. The presence of multiple forms of UDP-glucuronosyltransferases in the liver make this an unreliable method for studying glucuronidation in general.

7.3.4.2 Urinary 6β-hydroxycortisol (6β-OHC)

6β-Hydroxycortisol is produced from cortisol primarily by the hepatic mixed-function oxidase system (primarily, but not exclusively, by CYP3A). This is normally a minor pathway in the excretion of glucocorticoids, the major pathway being via 17-hydroxycorticosteroids (17-OHCS). Therefore the proportion of glucocorticoids excreted as the 6β-hydroxyderivatives should give a measure of the activity of CYP3A. A ratio of 6β-OHC/17-OHCS is a better indicator of changes in hepatic drug metabolism in man than the simple measurement of 6β-OHC excretion. The excretion of 6β-hydroxycortisol is not, however, a general indicator of hepatic drug-metabolising capacity as metabolite ratio studies with debrisoquine (see above) do not correlate with excretion of 6β-hydroxycortisol and there is also no correlation between excretion of 6β-hydroxycortisol and antipyrine clearance. This is due to different forms of cytochrome P450 in the liver being responsible for debrisoquine, antipyrine and cortisol metabolism. This test should only be used in a comparison of different groups of subjects and not as a predictive test of inter-individual variations in drug metabolism. 6β-Hydroxycortisol excretion also does not seem to be of use in assessing inhibition of drug metabolism.

The non-invasive methods of assessing drug metabolism are, therefore, of limited use in certain circumstances but are not of general applicability.

7.3.5 *In vivo/in vitro* correlations of drug metabolism

In the study of human drug metabolism one problem has become topical: the relationship between drug clearance measured *in vivo* (i.e. in the whole organism) and drug metabolism measured *in vitro* (i.e. in cells or fractions of tissues removed from the patient). This becomes relevant when it is known that the drug is predominantly cleared by hepatic metabolism. It is obviously much better to be able to check a patient's hepatic metabolism by a simple blood or urine test rather than by requiring a sample of liver tissue to examine the metabolism of the drug. The question becomes, how can one extrapolate data obtained from *in vitro* experiments to the whole organism?

As noted above, the measurement of urinary excretion of drugs has been shown to be a valid indicator of hepatic drug metabolism in certain circumstances, notably the metabolism of the model drugs antipyrine, debrisoquine and sparteine. Antipyrine is metabolised by the liver to three main metabolites. All of these metabolites are also found in the urine of patients given antipyrine. A study of the relative proportions of each metabolite formed by isolated liver tissue and found in the urine showed a very good correlation. A direct comparison of the *in vivo* clearance of antipyrine metabolites with *in vitro* assessment of hepatic drug metabolism in the same patient gave good correlation for all three metabolites. In this example, therefore, *in vivo* clearance is directly related to the ability of the liver to metabolise the drug. It is also possible to calculate scaling factors from such experiments such that enzyme activities in subcellular fractions (measured in, say, pmoles product formed/min/mg protein) can be used to calculate how fast a 70 kg man would clear the drug. For instance, using a bank of 15 human liver microsomal samples and the probe substrates phenytoin, tolbutamide, ibuprofen and diclofenac, the K_m and V_{max} values (and, thus, the intrinsic hepatic clearance ($Cl_{int} = V_{max}/K_m$)) can be found experimentally. Scaling these values to the intact human and comparing the values with published Cl_{int} values from *in vivo* experiments gives a reasonable correlation, particularly if albumin binding of the drugs *in vivo* is taken into account.

In other studies, the *in vivo* clearance of antipyrine has been shown to be unrelated to the *in vitro* metabolism of the precarcinogen, benzo[*a*]pyrene. This is not surprising as the two compounds are metabolised by different forms of cytochrome P450 in the human liver.

In the study of human drug metabolism, therefore, *in vivo* clearance values need to be interpreted carefully and not considered as directly related to drug metabolism in all cases – for instance, clearance may be purely by excretion of the parent compound as in the case of benzylpenicillin. *In vitro* data on the actual rate of probe substrate metabolism in either cells, slices or subcellular fractions, however, can be used to estimate intrinsic hepatic clearance in the whole body using appropriate scaling factors. These provisos should be borne in mind when discussing such *in vivo* and *in vitro* data.

There are methods available, therefore, for the study of hepatic drug metabolism in man. In order to put these methods into perspective, a number of examples of their use in the study of human drug metabolism will be given. It is hoped that the following examples will highlight the relevance of the study of drug metabolism in man in deciding how best to use the drugs to get the required effects without any toxic reaction to the drug.

7.4 CLINICAL RELEVANCE OF DRUG METABOLISM

As we have seen, drug metabolism is a major determinant of the change in drug concentration in the body and, thus, greatly affects the intensity and duration of action of drugs by altering the amount of the drug at its site of action. We have also seen how various methods can be used to measure drug metabolism in man. In this section we shall be looking at some examples of drug metabolism in a clinical context: how differences in drug metabolism – caused by genetic differences (pharmacogenetics), age factors, induction and inhibition, various diseases and dietary factors – can affect the way in which drugs act and how the methods discussed above can be used clinically in the assessment of drug-metabolising capacity of the liver and, thus, assist the clinician in deciding if there is a link between the actions or toxicity of the drug and its metabolism.

7.4.1 Effects of disease

Hepatic metabolism of drugs can be affected by many diseases, most of which, logically, are diseases of the liver (see Chapter 4). Early studies showed that cirrhosis of the liver caused a marked decrease in clearance of drugs from plasma but that the effects were mainly seen in phase 1 metabolism unless severe cirrhosis was examined. For instance, glucuronidation of lorazepam, oxazepam, morphine and paracetamol are unaffected in cirrhosis. Antipyrine clearance, however, a commonly used marker of phase 1 hepatic drug metabolism, has been shown to be reduced in chronic liver disease. In severe, uncompensated cirrhosis more enzyme activities are seen to be affected, including the glucuronidation of morphine, oxazepam and paracetamol. The difference in effect on phase 1 and 2 metabolism is, therefore, more one of degree. Chronic liver diseases seem to have marked substrate variation in their effects on hepatic drug metabolism. This has been emphasised in later studies looking at the clearance of antipyrine, aminopyrine, diazepam and indocyanine green (ICG) in the same patients. Four groups of patients were used: control, healthy volunteers, patients with hepatocellular diseases, and patients with hepatic carcinomas or cholestasis. Antipyrine clearance was measured employing the saliva test, aminopyrine and diazepam metabolism were measured using the breath tests, and indocyanine green was measured in plasma samples. It is known that antipyrine, aminopyrine and diazepam are cleared from the body mainly by hepatic metabolism and have a low extraction ratio (i.e. clearance is directly related to metabolism). Indocyanine green is not metabolised, and clearance is related to hepatic blood flow. Results obtained in the above study are shown in Table 7.7. It can be seen that the clearance of each drug is decreased by both hepatocellular diseases and hepatic carcinoma to a similar extent for each drug, whereas in cholestasis the elimination of antipyrine and ICG

Table 7.7 Effects of liver disease on clearance of drugs in man

Patient group	Aminopyrine	Diazepam	Antipyrine	Indocyanine green (ICG)
Control	100 ± 21[a]	100 ± 21	103 ± 36	98 ± 31
Hepatocellular diseases	38 ± 21	56 ± 18	45 ± 27	44 ± 24
Hepatic carcinoma	57 ± 22	69 ± 35	62 ± 37	66 ± 24
Cholestasis	110 ± 34	120 ± 42	64 ± 14	70 ± 23

Results expressed as % vs control.
[a] mean $\pm$ (standard deviation)
(Adapted from Vessell, E.S. (1980) *Proc. Natl. Acad. Sci. USA* **77**, 600–603. Used with permission of the author.)

Table 7.8 Usefulness of clearance of various drugs in assessing liver disease

Test	Percentage outside normal range	
	Hepatocellular diseases	Hepatic neoplasia
Aminopyrine	94	67
Diazepam	31	18
Antipyrine	24	20
ICG	69	22

(Adapted from Vessell, E.S. (1980) *Proc. Natl. Acad. Sci. USA* **77**, 600–603. Used with permission of the author.)

was markedly depressed but that of aminopyrine and diazepam were unaltered. Complex statistical analysis of these results gave the conclusion that it is misleading to extrapolate pharmacokinetic data from one drug to another even though it is thought that both drugs are cleared by the same mechanism (e.g. aminopyrine and antipyrine are cleared predominantly by hepatic metabolism but show opposite effects on clearance in cholestasis, whereas antipyrine and ICG are cleared by different mechanisms but show the same effect in cholestasis). This study also shows the relevance of the test applied to the prediction of altered hepatic function in the various disease states studied. All tests indicate a reduction in hepatic clearance in both hepatocellular and neoplastic diseases, but the aminopyrine breath test seems to be the best at discriminating between control and diseased liver states (Table 7.8).

Benzodiazepine metabolism in cirrhosis has been studied more extensively. Diazepam itself has been the subject of many studies that have shown marked changes in pharmacokinetics in liver disease. Liver diseases (hepatitis and cirrhosis) increase the half-life and decrease the clearance of diazepam. In patients without liver disease, diazepam half-life increases with multiple dosing due to accumulation of a metabolite, desmethyldiazepam, which apparently inhibits diazepam clearance. In cirrhotic patients the half-life of diazepam is unaffected by repeat dosing, probably due to the lower amount of metabolite formed leading to less product inhibition of the enzyme. These data suggest that diazepam will have a longer than expected effect in normal patients after multiple dosing but that this dosage regimen will have little effect on cirrhotic patients, although they will already show a much more marked effect of diazepam due to the impaired metabolism. It might be argued that in normal patients a steadily decreasing dose of diazepam is necessary to maintain plasma concentrations whereas in cirrhotic patients a lower but constant dose is needed. The changes in metabolism of benzodiazepines are also linked to the increased possibility of drug-induced coma in patients treated with these drugs who also have liver diseases. Impairment of psychomotor function has also been seen.

Using excretion of 7-hydroxycoumarin following a dose of coumarin (a marker of CYP2A6-dependent drug oxidation in the liver), it has been shown that hepatitis A infection severely curtails clearance of this drug (Figure 7.13).

Changes in hepatic drug clearance also occur in other diseases not directly affecting the liver, such as hormonal disorders of the thyroid and pituitary (e.g. hypothyroidism, dwarfism and acromegaly) and diabetes mellitus. Thyroid hormones generally stimulate hepatic drug metabolism and, therefore, hypothyroidism leads to diminished clearance of antipyrine, paracetamol and oxazepam, whereas hyperthyroidism gives increased antipyrine and oxazepam clearance. The effects of the diseases could be reversed by normalising the thyroid hormone levels. Pituitary dwarfism and acromegaly are lack of, and excess of, growth hormone, respectively. Growth hormone inhibits drug metabolism, particularly in children. Insulin, the hormone missing in some forms of diabetes mellitus, has recently been implicated

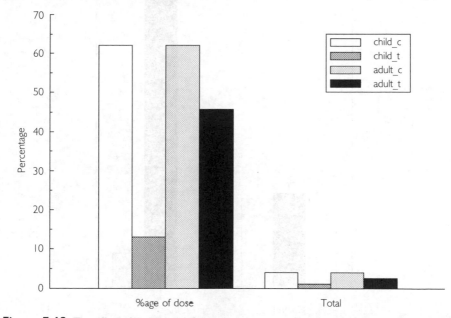

Figure 7.13 The effect of hepatitis A infection on clearance of total and 0–2 h percentage of dose of 7-hydroxycoumarin in children and adults. Child_c = control children; child_t = infected children; adult_c = control adult; adult_t = infected adult. (Data taken from Pasanen, M. et al. (1997) *Toxicology* **123**, 177–184. Used with permission of the authors and Elsevier Science.)

as an inducer of drug metabolism and lack of this hormone, therefore, leads to a reduced capacity of the liver to metabolise drugs. Such an effect has been reported for paracetamol glucuronidation in uncontrolled diabetics but not for oxazepam clearance. The effect on paracetamol metabolism was again reversed by treatment with insulin. Paradoxically, paracetamol clearance in obese patients (a condition often associated with type 2 diabetes mellitus) was increased over controls. This illustrates the difficulty of trying to decipher the effects of various changes on drug metabolism in the human population.

In one instance the relevance of the change in drug metabolism in a disease state is obvious and that is the alteration in primaquine clearance in patients suffering from malaria. In the case of primaquine, this drug is activated by phase 1 metabolism to become a potent antimalarial agent but the immune response to the malarial

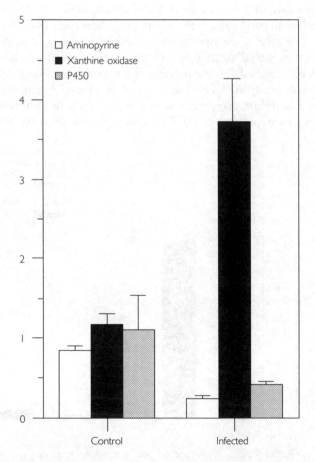

Figure 7.14 The effect of *Listeria monocytogenes* infection on aminopyrine *N*-demethylase (mmol HCHO/h), cytochrome P450 (nmol/mg protein) and xanthine oxidase (nmol/mg protein/min) in livers of mice. Data taken from Azri and Renton (1991) *Int. J. Immunopharm.* **13**, 197–204. Used with permission of Elsevier Science.

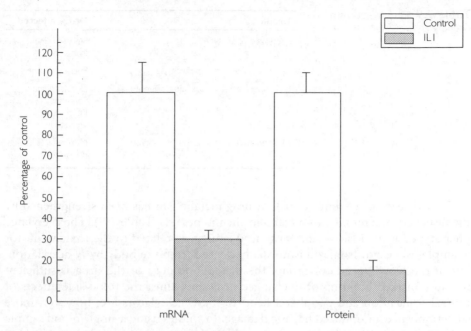

Figure 7.15 Effect of interleukin-1β (IL-1) treatment on cytochrome P450 2C11 mNRA and protein in isolated rat hepatocytes. (Data taken from Sewer, M. and Morgan, E.T. (1997) *Biochem. Pharmacol.* **54**, 729–737. Used with permission of the authors and Elsevier Science.)

parasite reduces the liver's ability to perform this activation and, thus, the disease itself reduces the effectiveness of the drug treatment of that disease. This is a manifestation of a more general phenomenon of decreased drug clearance in patients with infectious diseases. It is becoming clear that viral, bacterial and parasitic infections, which activate the immune system, cause a decrease in drug metabolism (Figure 7.14). This appears to be due to the effects on cytokines such as interleukin (IL)-1β on the liver. In the rat, treatment of hepatocytes with IL-β in culture led to a marked fall in CYP2C11 protein and mRNA (Figure 7.15). Nitric oxide (NO) did not, however, have any effect.

Disease states are, thus, a major influence on the ability of the body to clear drugs by metabolism and the altered drug metabolism in disease states may be of importance in the treatment of these diseases.

7.4.2 Genetic polymorphism in human drug metabolism

A genetic factor in determining the often large inter-individual variations in drug metabolism in man has been suspected for a long time since the metabolism of antipyrine in homozygous twins (identical twins) was shown to be almost the same, whereas in heterozygous (fraternal) twins there was as much variation as in the general population.

Table 7.9 Drug metabolism
phenotypes

Group	Drugs affected
Acetylator phenotype	Sulfadimidine Isoniazid
Pseudocholinesterase phenotype	Succinylcholine
Debrisoquine 4-hydroxylation phenotype	Debrisoquine Sparteine Phenacetin Guanoxan
Mephenytoin hydroxylation phenotype	Mephenytoin Phenytoin

The existence of genetic control of drug metabolism has been strengthened by the discovery of a number of metabolic phenotypes (see Table 7.9). The acetylator phenotypes, named 'slow' and 'fast' acetylators, are related to the toxicity of, for example, isoniazid. Isoniazid is normally cleared from the body by N-acetylation, but in the 'slow' acetylator group, the therapeutic dose of the drug is sufficient to cause marked build-up of unchanged drug and, thus, the toxic side effects of central stimulation and peripheral neuritis. 'Fast' acetylators are, however, more susceptible to drug-induced hepatic damage. In studies using a single blood sample following oral isoniazid treatment, over half of the subjects tested showed 'slow' acetylator status. The high incidence of the recessive trait indicates a selective advantage for the 'slow' acetylators which is not related to drug metabolism. It has been found that only one form of N-acetyltransferase (NAT2) is affected in the 'slow' acetylator and that other compounds cleared by acetylation (e.g. 4-amino-salicylate) are not affected as they are metabolised by NAT1. Multiple mutations of the NAT2 gene have been isolated and cloned.

The most common test for acetylator status is the acetylation of sulfadimidine which can be used to type a patient before isoniazid is given. The likely side effects of the drug will then be known. Interaction with other drugs can also be predicted, as 'slow' acetylators develop toxicity when isoniazid and phenytoin are given together, probably due to the higher blood levels of isoniazid inhibiting phenytoin metabolism, thus giving phenytoin toxicity. In these cases, knowing the acetylator status of the patient, toxicity can be avoided by modifying the dose of the drugs.

Pseudocholinesterase phenotype is characterised by a marked sensitivity to the muscle relaxant succinylcholine, which is normally metabolised by the serum pseudocholinesterase. Succinylcholine is of particular use in conjunction with general anaesthetics, tetanic seizures and in electroconvulsive therapy because of its extremely short half-life (about 2 min). Patients with an atypical pseudocholin-esterase, however, show a half-life of effect of the drug of about 2–3 hours. Total paralysis (including the respiratory muscles) for this length of time is obviously not advisable. The atypical reaction to succinylcholine has been shown to be con-trolled by an autosomal recessive gene and to be related to a structurally altered pseudocholinesterase in serum. The enzyme is not absent as in some other inherited defects of metabolism but is sufficiently altered to make it unable to metabolise

Table 7.10 Urinary excretion patterns of debrisoquine

Metabolite	Percentage dose excreted as metabolite			
	Subject 1	Subject 2	Subject 3	Subject 4
Debrisoquine	45	28	27	40
4-Hydroxydebrisoquine	30	37	39	2
Others	2.7	4.8	13.7	5.3

(Data from R.L. Smith, personal communication.)

succinylcholine. About 1 in every 3000 individuals will have atypical pseudocholinesterase and this can be tested by inhibition studies on the serum enzyme. The rarity of the recessive trait suggests that little selective advantage can be gained from having the atypical pseudocholinesterase.

Another atypical pseudocholinesterase has also been found with a higher activity towards succinylcholine. This is a very rare occurrence and again appears to be genetically controlled. The presence of this highly active pseudocholinesterase confers succinylcholine resistance on the individual.

Debrisoquine (once used in the treatment of hypertension) is metabolised by the liver mixed-function oxidase system mainly to 4-hydroxydebrisoquine. The enzyme responsible is CYP2D6. Marked inter-individual variation in excretion pattern and pharmacological effect of the drug was noted with maintenance doses ranging from 20–400 mg/day and urinary excretion of 8–70% as unchanged drug. A good correlation between dose needed and unchanged drug excreted was seen. Investigation of the metabolite pattern in the urine of volunteers given debrisoquine gave a clue to the nature of the variation (Table 7.10). One subject (no. 4) had a very low conversion of parent drug to the 4-hydroxyderivative. This subject was also very sensitive to the anti-hypertensive effects of debrisoquine. A larger study based on this chance finding revealed that there were, indeed, two populations of debrisoquine metabolisers and they could be classified according to the ratio of % dose excreted as debrisoquine:% dose excreted as 4-hydroxydebrisoquine. The major section of the population had a low ratio (about 1) and were termed 'extensive metabolisers' (EM); a much smaller section, with high ratios (about 20), were termed 'poor metabolisers' (PM). Over 90% belonged to the EM group. Family

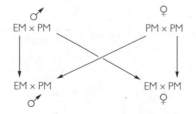

Figure 7.16 Family study of debrisoquine 4-hydroxylation. EM is extensive-metaboliser gene (dominant); PM is poor-metaboliser gene (recessive). (Data from R.L. Smith, personal communication.)

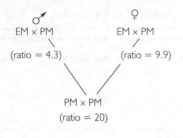

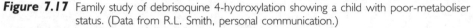

Figure 7.17 Family study of debrisoquine 4-hydroxylation showing a child with poor-metaboliser status. (Data from R.L. Smith, personal communication.)

studies indicated that extensive metabolism is the dominant trait. The genetic control is via a single gene pair, i.e. the offspring of a homozygous EM and a homozygous PM will all be heterozygous (Figure 7.16). All of the offspring will therefore be extensive metabolisers. Two heterozygous parents can produce a homozygous recessive child and this has been seen in practice (see Figure 7.17). It should be noted that heterozygous extensive metabolisers have higher ratios than homozygotes, indicating that the dominance of the extensive trait is not complete. Extensive research has identified a whole family of aberrant CYP2D6 genes, some coding for enzyme with reduced activity, some for protein with no activity and some that do not produce any product (null mutations). One set of mutations (with one loss of function mutation which terminates the protein after 181 amino acids instead of the wild type 497) represents 65% of PM status individuals.

We therefore have a drug oxidation polymorphism that can relatively easily be measured by examining the metabolite ratio of debrisoquine in urine. This would be merely of academic interest, however, if it were not for the fact that the debrisoquine polymorphism turns out to be a model for many other clinically used drugs where a genetic component controlling the drug metabolism has been suspected. A list of drugs whose metabolism is associated with debrisoquine 4-hydroxylation is shown in Table 7.11. The list is expanding rapidly and debrisoquine 4-hydroxylation may be a very good model drug for a test of metabolic status. Not all genetic control of drug metabolism, however, is similar to that of debrisoquine: the metabolism of mephenytoin is also genetically regulated but is not associated with the debrisoquine polymorphism. Indeed, it is thought that another isoform of

Table 7.11 Drugs whose metabolism is related to debrisoquine 4-hydroxylation

Nortryptiline	Metoprolol
Phenacetin	4-Methoxyamphetamine
Phenformin	Carbocysteine
Phenytoin	Bufurolol
Sparteine	Encainide
Perhexiline	Guanoxan
Metiamide	

Table 7.12 The effect of debrisoquine phenotype on the metabolism of guanoxan

| Phenotype | % dose excreted as | | Ratio $\left(\dfrac{\text{parent drug}}{\text{metabolite}}\right)$ |
	Guanoxan	OH-guanoxan	
EM	1.5 ± 0.3[a]	29 ± 5	0.06 ± 0.02
PM	48 ± 12	6.2 ± 1.4	7.8 ± 0.2

[a] Mean ± (standard deviation)
(Data from R.L. Smith, personal communication.)

cytochrome P450 is involved, namely CYP2C19. Again, as with CYP2D6, the major mutant CYP2C19 gene leads to a truncated non-functional protein.

The genetic polymorphisms discussed above could be the explanation for a number of unexplained sensitive groups of individuals, e.g. unusual sensitivity to phenytoin where sensitive individuals develop toxic side effects (e.g. nystagmus and ataxia) at much lower doses of the drug. This sensitivity is related to reduced 4-hydroxylation of phenytoin and has now been tentatively correlated with the poor metaboliser status of mephenytoin.

Phenacetin metabolism is thought to be related to debrisoquine metaboliser status. In some patients, phenacetin is hydroxylated rather than the usual route of de-ethylation. This unusual route of metabolism was thought to be the cause of the toxic side effects seen (methaemoglobinaemia). Impaired metabolism of phenacetin to paracetamol, and subsequent conversion of the remaining phenacetin to the 2-hydroxylated products, is correlated to poor metaboliser status for debrisoquine.

The metabolism of guanoxan is also correlated with debrisoquine 4-hydroxylation so that poor metabolisers of debrisoquine are also poor metabolisers of guanoxan (Table 7.12). Guanoxan is, like debrisoquine, an antihypertensive and has side effects similar to debrisoquine – poor metabolisers are, therefore, more susceptible to the central effects and hepatotoxicity of guanoxan.

The simple debrisoquine or mephenytoin metabolite ratio test can therefore be used as a routine test for susceptibility of patients to the toxic effects of a number of clinically important drugs, and it has useful predictive value in this respect. Using these tests it has been shown that different racial groups exhibit different proportions of poor and extensive metabolisers (Table 7.13). Egyptians show the lowest incidence of debrisoquine 'poor metaboliser' status (about 1%) whereas

Table 7.13 Incidence of 'poor'-metaboliser (PM) phenotype in different ethnic groups

Ethnic group	Number studied	Number PM	Percentage incidence of PM
Caucasian	106	5	5
Egyptian	72	1	1.5
Nigerian	34	5	15
Ghanian	27	3	12

(Data from R.L. Smith, personal communication.)

West Africans show a high incidence (about 13%). Caucasians are intermediate between these two groups. For mephenytoin 'poor metaboliser' status, 2.7% of Caucasians and 18% of Japanese show this trait. This is a good example from the developing discipline of ethnopharmacology.

The existence of at least two sub-populations with markedly different drug metabolising capacities has far-reaching and important correlates, particularly where drug oxidation is concerned and especially considering the high incidence of individuals with impaired drug oxidising capacity. From the examples given above, it becomes obvious that drugs linked to the debrisoquine or mephenytoin phenotype should be given in lower doses to PM individuals than to EM, so reducing the risk of overdose and subsequent toxic effects. It is, in fact, possible that drugs have been withdrawn from clinical use due to a high incidence of toxic side effects, when a reduction in dosage after a debrisoquine test may have been all that was required. Phenformin, for example, has been restricted due to build-up of lactic acid (lactoacidosis) in certain individuals. Phenformin metabolism is known to be correlated to debrisoquine 4-hydroxylation but no information is available as to whether lactoacidosis is correlated to PM status. If such a correlation was found, phenformin could be reintroduced on a wider scale following a debrisoquine test of prospective recipients. Indeed, a volunteer panel of known EM/PM-status people is routinely used in the pharmaceutical industry to enable them to investigate the effect of debrisoquine metabolism status on the effects of their compounds under test. Typing of liver cells and slices in tissue banks is also now routinely performed and samples of known genetic status can be ordered for experimentation.

7.4.3 Induction and inhibition of drug metabolism

In Chapter 3 it was seen that the enzymes involved in drug metabolism can be induced or inhibited by a wide variety of compounds, from the drug metabolised by a particular enzyme to a food component or tobacco smoke. These effects can, of course, also be seen in man and are of great importance in determining such things as drug interactions and the effects of diet on drug metabolism. Some examples of these interactions are given below.

The use of multiple drug therapy in the treatment of many diseases has led to problems with drug interactions. Many drug interactions are the result of interference of one drug with the metabolism of another and the subsequent increase or

Table 7.14 Drugs which interact with phenobarbitone on a metabolic level

Phenytoin	Chlorpromazine
Warfarin	Phenylbutazone
Bishydroxycoumarin	Pethidine
Lignocaine	Cyclophosphamide
Digitoxin	Griseofulvin
Fenoprofen	Cortisol
DDT	

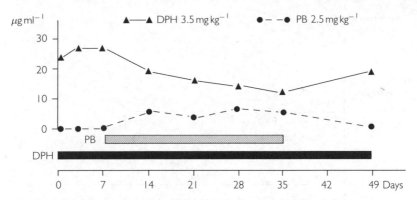

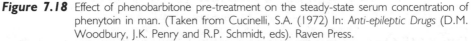

Figure 7.18 Effect of phenobarbitone pre-treatment on the steady-state serum concentration of phenytoin in man. (Taken from Cucinelli, S.A. (1972) In: *Anti-epileptic Drugs* (D.M. Woodbury, J.K. Penry and R.P. Schmidt, eds). Raven Press.

decrease in the clearance of the latter drug. Interaction of drugs with phenobarbitone is, perhaps, the most studied example of this phenomenon as phenobarbitone is an inducer of the metabolism of many other drugs (see Chapter 3) and numerous clinical interactions with this drug are seen. Table 7.14 lists some of the drugs that interact with phenobarbitone at a metabolic level. Of particular interest is the interaction of phenobarbitone and phenytoin that are both used in the treatment of epilepsy. Treatment of patients already given phenytoin with phenobarbitone reduced the steady state serum concentration of phenytoin markedly (Figure 7.18). Withdrawal of phenobarbitone treatment returned serum concentrations of phenytoin to control levels. Control of seizures by phenytoin can thus be greatly influenced by the presence of phenobarbitone, itself a drug used to control seizure. The complex interactions theoretically available make the use of phenytoin and phenobarbitone in combination a somewhat unpredictable and therefore dangerous therapy.

The interaction of phenobarbitone with digitoxin (a drug with low therapeutic index) is also of major concern to the clinician. Digitoxin is a cardiac glycoside used in the treatment of heart failure, but with major side effects at slightly above clinical doses (toxicity includes anorexia, CNS disturbances, atrial fibrillation and tachycardia). Steady state concentrations of digitoxin fell to about half following treatment with phenobarbitone, with a marked fall in plasma half-life of digitoxin from about 8 to 4 days. Polar metabolites of digitoxin increased in urine following phenobarbitone treatment. It thus appears that phenobarbitone increased the metabolism of digitoxin, thereby reducing its serum concentration and effectiveness. Increasing the dose of digitoxin to counter this effect will lead to excess, toxic concentrations of digitoxin being present in serum when phenobarbitone is withdrawn (Figure 7.19). A very similar effect is seen with warfarin (this has been discussed in Chapter 3). The use of phenobarbitone to increase drug-metabolising capacity in liver diseases has been attempted. For instance patients with liver disease metabolise phenylbutazone very slowly (plasma $t_{1/2}$ of about 100 h) and this can be shortened to about 50–55 h by treatment with phenobarbitone.

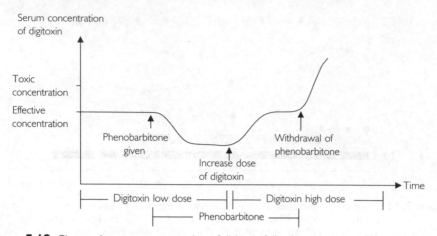

Figure 7.19 Changes in serum concentration of digitoxin following treatment with, and withdrawal of, phenobarbitone.

Patients suffering from unconjugated hyperbilirubinaemia (caused by a relative deficiency of UDP-glucuronosyltransferase in the liver, whether the mild Gilbert's disease or the more severe Crigler–Najjar syndrome) can be treated with phenobarbitone to relieve the symptoms. Dramatic reductions in serum bilirubin levels can easily be achieved by this method, which relies on the ability of phenobarbitone to induce hepatic UDP-glucuronosyltransferase activity as there is a linear relationship between hepatic UDP-glucuronosyltransferase activity and bilirubin clearance. Other barbiturates such as barbitone, hexobarbitone and amylobarbitone show similar effects to phenobarbitone and should, perhaps, be viewed as a group.

Of the other drugs that are considered to be inducers of drug metabolism, the majority are seen to induce their own metabolism. Tolerance to glutethimide, meprobamate and diazepam, for instance, develops partly due to the increased metabolism of the drug owing to induction. Carbamazepine is a drug investigated in terms of induction of metabolism of itself, other exogenous compounds and endogenous compounds. The clearance of antipyrine, measured by the saliva test, increased after two weeks' treatment while carbamazepine half-life, measured in plasma, decreased from a control level of 32.3 h to 19.1 h during the same period. Increases in enzymes involved in endogenous metabolism were also found in this study, with 6β-hydroxylation of cortisol increased, and the level of leucocyte δ-aminolevulinic acid synthetase (the rate-limiting enzyme in the biosynthesis of haem) also increased. Carbamazepine has also been shown to induce the metabolism of phenytoin and warfarin.

Oral contraceptives containing estrogens and/or progestins have been reported to inhibit hepatic drug metabolism, probably by competitive inhibition. Steroids are metabolised in the liver by the same enzyme systems as drugs and therefore such inhibitory interactions are not unlikely. Aminopyrine clearance is significantly lower in women taking an oral contraceptive pill but there is no effect on paracetamol clearance.

Another compound known to affect drug metabolism is ethanol, which again shares a common breakdown enzyme with drugs and steroids. Ethanol may act acutely to inhibit drug metabolism but in the longer term as an inducer of cytochrome P450 2E1. Co-administration of ethanol with certain drugs can, therefore, enhance the effect of the drug by leading to a slower clearance. This is part of the problem associated with the enhanced action of benzodiazepines when taken with ethanol. The habitual drinker, however, may have an enhanced drug metabolising capacity – the CYP2E1 induction caused by ethanol is a defence mechanism of the body as this form is the one that metabolises ethanol (also known as the microsomal ethanol oxidising system, see Chapter 1). CYP2E1 can also metabolise paracetamol, isoniazid and carcinogenic amines. The interaction with paracetamol is thought to lead to an enhanced toxicity of the analgesic by increasing the formation of the toxic metabolite of the drug.

Also of great clinical relevance is the induction of the phase 1 cytochrome P450-dependent metabolism of cyclosporine. Cyclosporine is used in the prevention of rejection following kidney transplantation and induction of the metabolising enzyme, leading to extensive metabolism of the drug, can lead to failure of the drug to prevent rejection of the graft.

It can be seen from these examples that drug–drug interactions involving induction or inhibition of drug metabolism can be of great importance in determining the action and toxicity of drugs.

Induction and inhibition are, however, important in another respect and that is the interaction of environmental factors with hepatic drug metabolism. One major group of compounds, widespread in our environment, which have a major effect on hepatic drug metabolism are the polycyclic hydrocarbons (e.g. benzo[a]pyrene). These are found in cigarette smoke and in any food cooked over open heat (e.g. charcoal-broiled meat). Much work has been done on the effects of polycyclic hydrocarbons on drug metabolism and the relationship to the intake of tobacco smoke and charcoal-broiled meat.

The clearance of antipyrine and paracetamol is greatly increased by smoking (Figure 7.20). It is seen that there is a graded response to the number of cigarettes

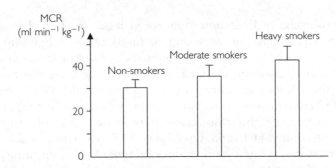

Figure 7.20 Relationship between daily cigarette consumption and clearance of antipyrine. MCR = mean clearance rate. (Taken from Vestal, R.E. et al. (1975) *Clin. Pharm. Ther.* **18**, 425–432.)

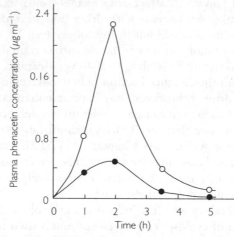

Figure 7.21 Mean plasma concentration of phenacetin in smokers (●) and non-smokers (○) as a function of time following oral administration of a 900 mg dose. (Taken from Pantuck, E. *et al.* (1972) *Science* **175**, 1248–1250. Used with permission of the author. © 1972 AAAS.)

smoked. The effect of cigarette smoking on the plasma concentrations of phenacetin is even more dramatic (Figure 7.21). The area under the concentration curve is seen to be much less in smokers, indicating that the bioavailability of phenacetin is lower, but the half-life is similar in both groups. Animal studies have shown that benzo[*a*]pyrene – a major constituent of tobacco smoke – induces mixed-function oxidase activity in the small intestine and the increased first-pass effect caused by such induction may be the explanation of the reduced bioavailability without increased hepatic metabolism seen in man. Benzo[*a*]pyrene is known to induce CYP1A1 and 1A2 in man and it is these forms that perform the enhanced metabolism seen in smokers. Other drugs, however, are unaffected by smoking with respect to their metabolism. In drug therapy it is therefore important to know the smoking habits of the patients, particularly if the drug to be used is metabolised by CYP1A1 or 1A2.

Looking at polycyclic hydrocarbon inducers in food, we find that any meat cooked over open heat (i.e. any browning of food) causes a build-up of such compounds. These have been shown to be potent inducers of drug metabolism in a very similar manner to cigarette smoking and, indeed, the same compounds are responsible for the effects (i.e. benzo[*a*]pyrene induction of CYP1A1 and 1A2). Plasma levels of phenacetin are markedly reduced in subjects on a charcoal-broiled meat diet – the subjects in this case acting as their own controls, so reducing problems from inter-individual variations (Table 7.15). As with tobacco smoking the area under the curve is significantly reduced (Figure 7.22) indicating a lack of bioavailability of phenacetin in subjects eating charcoal-broiled meat, probably because the inducers have increased enzyme activity in the small intestine so stopping uptake of the drug. It is seen that at least 75% of phenacetin never enters

Table 7.15 The effect of a diet containing charcoal-broiled meat on the plasma concentration of phenacetin in man

Time after administration (h)	Plasma phenacetin concentration (ng ml^{-1})	
	Control diet	Charcoal diet
1	1328 ± 481[a]	319 ± 90
2	925 ± 166	163 ± 32
3	313 ± 60	74 ± 17
4	149 ± 27	34 ± 9
5	66 ± 14	15 ± 4

[a] Mean ± (standard deviation)
(Data from Pantuck, E. et al. (1972) Science **175**, 1248–1250. Used with permission of the author. © 1972 AAAS.)

the plasma in subjects on a charcoal-broiled meat diet. This has obvious clinical relevance for treatment with this drug: a patient may need four times the dose to achieve the same effect simply because of eating charcoal-broiled meat.

If antipyrine and theophylline plasma half-life and clearance are examined in subjects on a charcoal-broiled meat diet a different picture emerges. For both antipyrine and theophylline, plasma half-life is decreased and total clearance increased. As antipyrine and theophylline are both predominantly cleared by hepatic metabolism, it seems reasonable to suggest that the effect of charcoal-broiled meat, in this instance, is on the liver and that we are seeing induction of hepatic mixed-function oxidases by the polycyclic hydrocarbons in the diet. This is similar to the effect of tobacco smoke seen earlier.

More recently, a fascinating story has emerged regarding the influence of grapefruit juice (but not other citrus fruit juices) on drug availability. The oral availability of many commonly used drugs such as felodipine, cyclosporine A, ethynylestradiol and nifedipine, has been shown to be markedly increased by a single glass of grapefruit juice and the common factor in the drugs seems to be their metabolism by CYP3A4, the major form in man. Early studies indicated that extracts of grapefruit juice could inhibit CYP3A4 in human liver microsomes and some studies even suggested that flavanoids (such as naringin) in the grapefruit juice were the active ingredients. More recent studies have suggested, however, that the mechanism of action of grapefruit juice may be quite different. Treatment of adult males with one glass of grapefruit juice per day for 8 days and subsequent analysis of biopsies of intestinal tissue, assay of felodipine clearance after oral dosing and assay of CYP3A4 in liver using the erythromycin breath test showed that liver CYP3A4 was unaffected, whereas felodipine pharmacokinetics were markedly altered and intestinal content of CYP3A4 was reduced by 62% (Figure 7.23). This suggests that first-pass metabolism of felodipine in the intestine is inhibited by grapefruit juice and not its metabolism by the liver. Work in rats has suggested that the content of flavanoids is too low in grapefruit juice to support the hypothesis that they are the active constituents. It is thought more likely that hydrophobic substances (maybe triterpene coumarins) are the active ingredients.

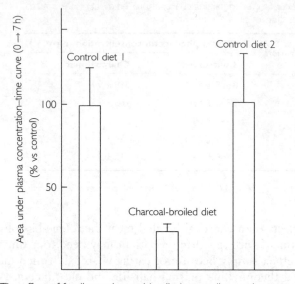

Figure 7.22 The effect of feeding a charcoal-broiled meat diet on the area-under-curve for phenacetin. (Taken from Pantuck, E. *et al.* (1972) *Science* **175**, 1248–1250. Used with permission of the author. © 1972 AAAS.)

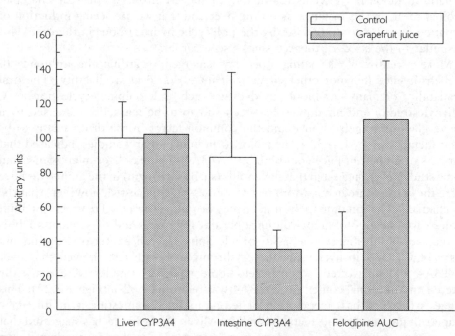

Figure 7.23 The effect of drinking grapefruit juice on liver and intestinal cytochrome P450 (CYP) 3A4 and felodipine bioavailability (AUC) in man. (Data taken from Lown *et al.* (1997) *J. Clin. Invest.* **99**, 2545–2553. Used with permission of the authors.)

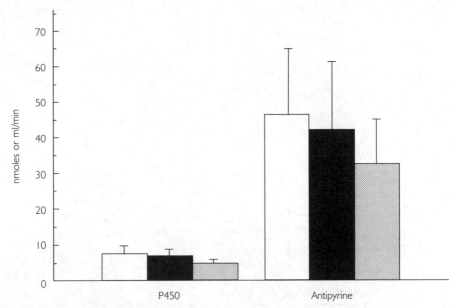

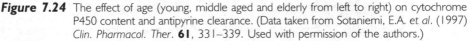

Figure 7.24 The effect of age (young, middle aged and elderly from left to right) on cytochrome P450 content and antipyrine clearance. (Data taken from Sotaniemi, E.A. *et al.* (1997) *Clin. Pharmacol. Ther.* **61**, 331–339. Used with permission of the authors.)

Induction and inhibition of drug metabolism, whether by other drugs, environmental or dietary chemicals, can be important factors in the action of drugs. Changes in metabolism caused by such factors should be taken into account when treating patients.

7.4.4 Age factors

The role of aging as a factor in drug-metabolising capacity has been a subject of debate with a number of opposing views. Is the perceived decrease in drug metabolism in old people (manifested as a slower clearance of drugs and an extended duration of action and enhanced effect) a reality or a consequence of slower metabolic rate or generally decreased liver capacity and lower blood flow? Some recent studies have shown that cytochrome P450 content does, indeed, drop in aged individuals (after 70 years of age) and that this correlates to a longer $t_{1/2}$ for antipyrine (Figure 7.24). Clearance of probe drugs metabolised by CYP3A4 (lignocaine *N*-deethylation) and CYP2A6 (coumarin 7-hydroxylation) was found to be reduced in older men and women (Figure 7.25). There is clearly some role for decreased drug metabolism in the noted slower clearance of drugs in the elderly.

7.5 SUMMARY

Using as a theoretical basis the mathematical interpretation of drug concentrations in the body and drug elimination from the body (i.e. pharmacokinetics), we can

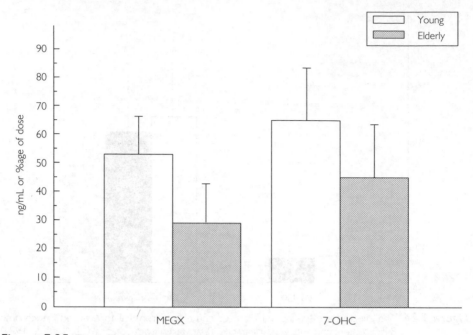

Figure 7.25 The effect of age on the metabolism of lignocaine to MEGX and coumarin to 7-hydroxy-coumarin in man. (Data taken from Sotaniemi, E.A. et al. (1996) *Thérapie* **51**, 363–366. Used with permission of the authors.)

measure various parameters of the drugs used in modern medicine. A more physiologically based assessment of pharmacokinetics can also be made using the newer models. These parameters (such as half-life, clearance, etc.) can be related to the duration and intensity of action of a drug to give a meaningful measure of a drug's usefulness and possible toxicity.

The methods used in measuring these parameters have been discussed and examples of how these methods can be used have been given. The clinical relevance of the examples chosen has been explained, where known.

It is hoped that this chapter has given some insight into the usefulness of pharmacokinetics and drug metabolic measurements in man but that, at the same time, it has also pointed out the disadvantages of the methods and, perhaps, stimulated some thought as to how these techniques could be improved or better used.

FURTHER READING

Books and symposia

Curry, S.H. and Whelpton, R. (1983) *Manual of Laboratory Pharmacokinetics*. Wiley, Chichester.

Hladky, S.B. (1990) *Pharmacokinetics*. Manchester University Press, Manchester.

Rowland, M. and Tozer, T.M. (1989) *Clinical Pharmacokinetics: Concepts and Applications*, 2nd edn. Lea and Febiger, Philadelphia.

Reviews and original articles

Alvan, G. (1991) Clinical consequences of polymorphic drug oxidation. *Fund. Clin. Pharmacol.* 5, 209–228.

Alvan, G. (1992) Genetic polymorphisms in drug metabolism. *J. Int. Med.* 231, 571–573.

Berry, M.N. *et al.* (1992) Techniques for pharmacological and toxicological studies with isolated hepatocyte preparations. *Life Sci.* 51, 1–16.

Berthou, F. *et al.* (1989) Comparison of caffeine metabolism by slices, microsomes and hepatocyte cultures from adult human liver. *Xenobiotica* 19, 410–417.

Brosen, K. (1990) Recent developments in hepatic drug oxidations. Implications for clinical pharmacokinetics. *Clin. Pharmacokin.* 18, 220–239.

Coeke, S. *et al.* (1998) Hormonal regulation of microsomal flavin-containing mono-oxygenase activity by sex steroids and growth hormone in co-cultured adult male rat hepatocytes. *Biochem. Pharmacol.* 56, 1047–1051.

Eichelbaum, M. and Gross, A.S. (1990) The genetic polymorphism of debrisoquine/sparteine metabolism – clinical aspects. *Pharmacol. Ther.* 46, 377–394.

Fabre, G. *et al.* (1990) Human hepatocytes as a key model to improve preclinical drug development. *Eur. J. Drug Metab. Pharmacokin.* 15, 165–171.

Fukuda, K. *et al.* (1997) Grapefruit component interacting with rat and human P450 CYP3A: possible involvement of non-flavanoid components in drug interaction. *Biol. Pharm. Bull.* 20, 560–564.

George, J. and Farrell, G.C. (1991) Role of human hepatic cytochromes P450 in drug metabolism and toxicity. *Aust. NZ J. Med.* 21, 356–362.

Gonzalez, F.J. and Meyer, U.A. (1991) Molecular genetics of the debrisoquine/sparteine polymorphism. *Clin. Pharmacol. Ther.* 50, 233–238.

Guttendorf, R.J. and Wedlund, P.J. (1992) Genetic aspects of drug disposition and therapeutics. *J. Clin. Pharmacol.* 32, 107–117.

Idle, J.R. and Smith, R.L. (1979) Polymorphisms of oxidation at carbon centres of drugs and their clinical significance. *Drug Metab. Rev.* 9, 301–318.

Kalow, W. and Tang, B.K. (1991) Caffeine as a metabolic probe: exploration of the enzyme-inducing effect of cigarette smoking. *Clin. Pharmacol. Ther.* 49, 44–48.

Kraul, H. *et al.* (1991) Comparison of *in vitro* and *in vivo* biotransformation in patients with liver disease of differing severity. *Eur. J. Clin. Pharmacol.* 41, 475–480.

Kroemer, H.K. and Klotz, U. (1992) Glucuronidation of drugs. *Clin. Pharmacokin.* 23, 292–310.

Ladona, M.G. *et al.* (1991) Differential foetal development of the O- and N-demethylation of codeine and dextromethorphan in man. *Br. J. Clin. Pharmacol.* 32, 295–302.

Lavrijsen, K. *et al.* (1992) Comparative metabolism of flunarizine in rats, dogs and man: an *in vitro* study with subcellular liver fractions and isolated hepatocytes. *Xenobiotica* 22, 815–836.

Loft, S. and Poulsen, H.E. (1990) Prediction of xenobiotic metabolism by non-invasive methods. *Pharmacol. Toxicol.* 67, 101–108.

Lou, Y.C. (1990) Differences in drug metabolism polymorphism between Orientals and Caucasians. *Drug Metab. Rev.* 22, 451–475.

Lown, K.S. *et al.* (1997) Grapefruit juice increases felodipine oral availability in humans by decreasing intestinal CYP3A protein expression. *J. Clin. Invest.* 99, 2545–2553.

Lucas, D. *et al.* (1990) Ethanol-inducible cytochrome P450: assessment of substrate specific chemical probes in rat liver microsomes. *Alcohol Clin. Exp. Res.* 14, 590–594.

Meyer, U.A. and Zanger, U.M. (1997) Molecular mechanisms of genetic polymorphisms of drug metabolism. *Ann. Rev. Pharmacol. Toxicol.* **37**, 269–296.

Moshage, H. and Yap, S.H. (1992) Primary cultures of human hepatocytes: a unique system for studies in toxicology, virology, parasitology and liver pathophysiology in man. *J. Hepatol.* **15**, 404–413.

Nagata, K. and Yamazoe, Y. (2000) Pharmacogenetics of sulfotransferase. *Ann. Rev. Pharmacol. Toxicol.* **40**, 159–176.

Osborne, N.J. *et al.* (1991) Interethnic differences in drug glucuronidation: a comparison of paracetamol metabolism in Causasian and Chinese. *Br. J. Clin. Pharmacol.* **32**, 765–767.

Paine, A.J. (1990) The maintenance of cytochrome P450 in rat hepatocyte cultures. Some applications of liver cell cultures to the study of drug metabolism, toxicity and the induction of the P450 system. *Chemico-Biol. Interact.* **74**, 1–31.

Park, B.K. (1981) Assessment of urinary 6β-hydroxycortisol as an *in vivo* index of mixed-function oxygenase activity. *Br. J. Clin. Pharmacol.* **12**, 97–102.

Pasanen, M. *et al.* (1997) Hepatitis A impairs the function of human hepatic CYP2A6 *in vivo*. *Toxicology* **123**, 177–184.

Sewer, M.B. and Morgan, E.T. (1997) Nitric oxide-independent suppression of P450 2C11 expression by interleukin-1β and endotoxin in primary rat hepatocytes. *Biochem. Pharmacol.* **54**, 729–737.

Smith, D.A. (1998) Human cytochromes P450: selectivity and measurement *in vivo*. *Xenobiotica* **28**, 1095–1128.

Smith, G. *et al.* (1998) Molecular genetics of the human cytochrome P450 monooxygenase superfamily. *Xenobiotica* **28**, 1129–1165.

Sotaniemi, E.A. *et al.* (1996) Age and CYP3A4 and CYP2A6 activities marked by the metabolism of lignocaine and coumarin in man. *Therapie* **51**, 363–366.

Sotaniemi, E.A. *et al.* (1997) Age and cytochrome P450-linked drug metabolism in humans: an analysis of 226 subjects with equal histopathologic conditions. *Clin. Pharmacol. Ther.* **61**, 331–339.

Srivastava, P. *et al.* (1991) Effect of Plasmodium berghei infection and chloroquine on the hepatic drug metabolising system of mice. *Int. J. Parasitol.* **4**, 463–466.

Tanaka, E. (1999) Update: genetic polymorphisms of drug-metabolising enzymes. *J. Clin. Pharm. Ther.* **24**, 323–329.

Tuckey, R.H. and Strassburg, C.P. (2000) Human UDP-glucuronosyltransferases: metabolism, expression and disease. *Ann. Rev. Pharmacol. Toxicol.* **40**, 581–616.

Van der Weide, J. and Steijns, L.S. (1999) Cytochrome P450 enzyme system: genetic polymorphisms and impact on clinical pharmacology. *Ann. Clin. Biochem.* **36**, 722–729.

Vessell, E.S. (1977) Genetic and environmental factors affecting drug disposition in man. *Clin. Pharmacol. Ther.* **22**, 659–679.

Watkins, P.B. *et al.* (1989) Erythromycin breath test as an assay of glucocorticoid-inducible liver cytochrome P450. *J. Clin. Invest.* **83**, 688.

Wrighton, S.A. and Stevens, J.C. (1992) The human hepatic cytochromes P450 involved in drug metabolism. *Crit. Rev. Toxicol.* **22**, 1–21.

Yasumore, T. *et al.* (1990) Polymorphism in hydroxylation of mephenytoin and hexobarbital stereoisomers in relation to hepatic P450 human-2. *Clin. Pharmacol. Ther.* **47**, 313–322.

A list of useful web sites is included at the end of Chapters 2 and 3.

INDEX

Page numbers in *italic* refer to tables